HEART-HEALTHY KITCHEN

Flavorful Recipes for A Healthy Heart

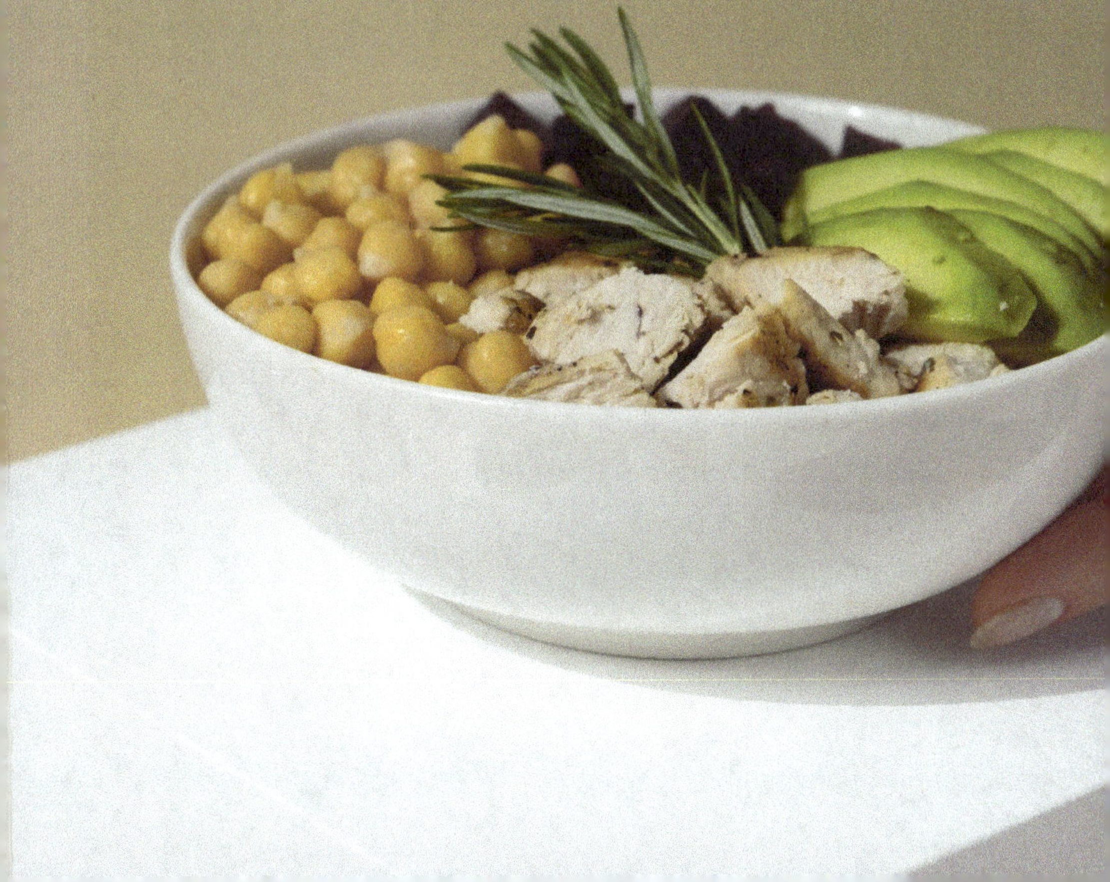

Contents

Dinner 38

Introduction

"Heart-Healthy Kitchen: Flavorful Recipes for a Healthy Heart" is a comprehensive guide to cooking delicious and nutritious meals that support cardiovascular wellness. Designed for anyone looking to maintain a healthy heart or improve their overall well-being, this book makes it easy to incorporate heart-friendly foods into your daily diet without sacrificing taste.

This book is ideal for anyone looking to improve their heart health through diet, whether they have been diagnosed with heart disease, have a family history of cardiovascular issues, or simply want to adopt healthier eating habits. It is also a valuable resource for caregivers, dietitians, and healthcare professionals who support individuals in managing their heart health. "Heart-Healthy Kitchen" is perfect for home cooks of all skill levels who want to prepare nutritious, heart-friendly meals for themselves and their loved ones.

Breakfast

Two-Ingredient Banana Pancakes

🍴 2 servings   🕐 15 minutes

INGREDIENTS

2 large eggs

1 medium banana

DIRECTIONS

1. Puree eggs and banana in a blender until smooth.

2. Lightly oil a large nonstick skillet (see Tip) and heat over medium heat. Using 2 tablespoons of batter for each pancake, drop 4 mounds of batter into the pan. Cook until bubbles appear on the surface and the edges look dry, 2 to 4 minutes. Using a thin spatula, gently flip the pancakes and cook until browned on the bottom, 1 to 2 minutes more. Transfer the pancakes to a plate. Lightly oil the pan again and repeat with the remaining batter.

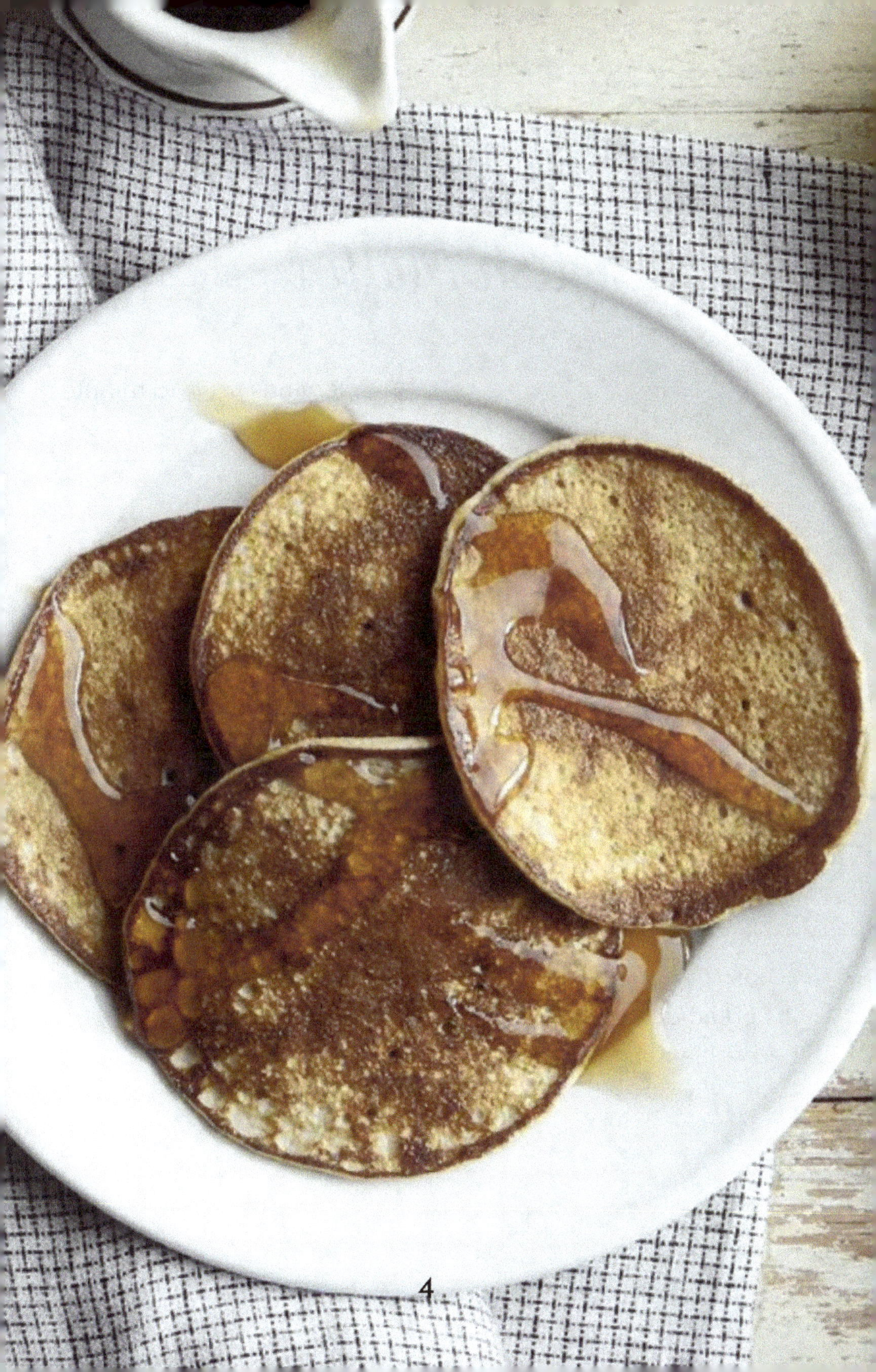

Peanut Butter & Chia Berry Jam English Muffin

🍴 2 servings   🕐 15 minutes

INGREDIENTS

½ cup unsweetened mixed frozen berries

2 teaspoons chia seeds

2 teaspoons natural peanut butter

1 whole-wheat English muffin, toasted

DIRECTIONS

1. Microwave berries in a medium microwave-safe bowl for 30 seconds; stir and microwave 30 seconds more. Stir in chia seeds.

2. Spread peanut butter on the English muffin. Top with the berry-chia mixture.

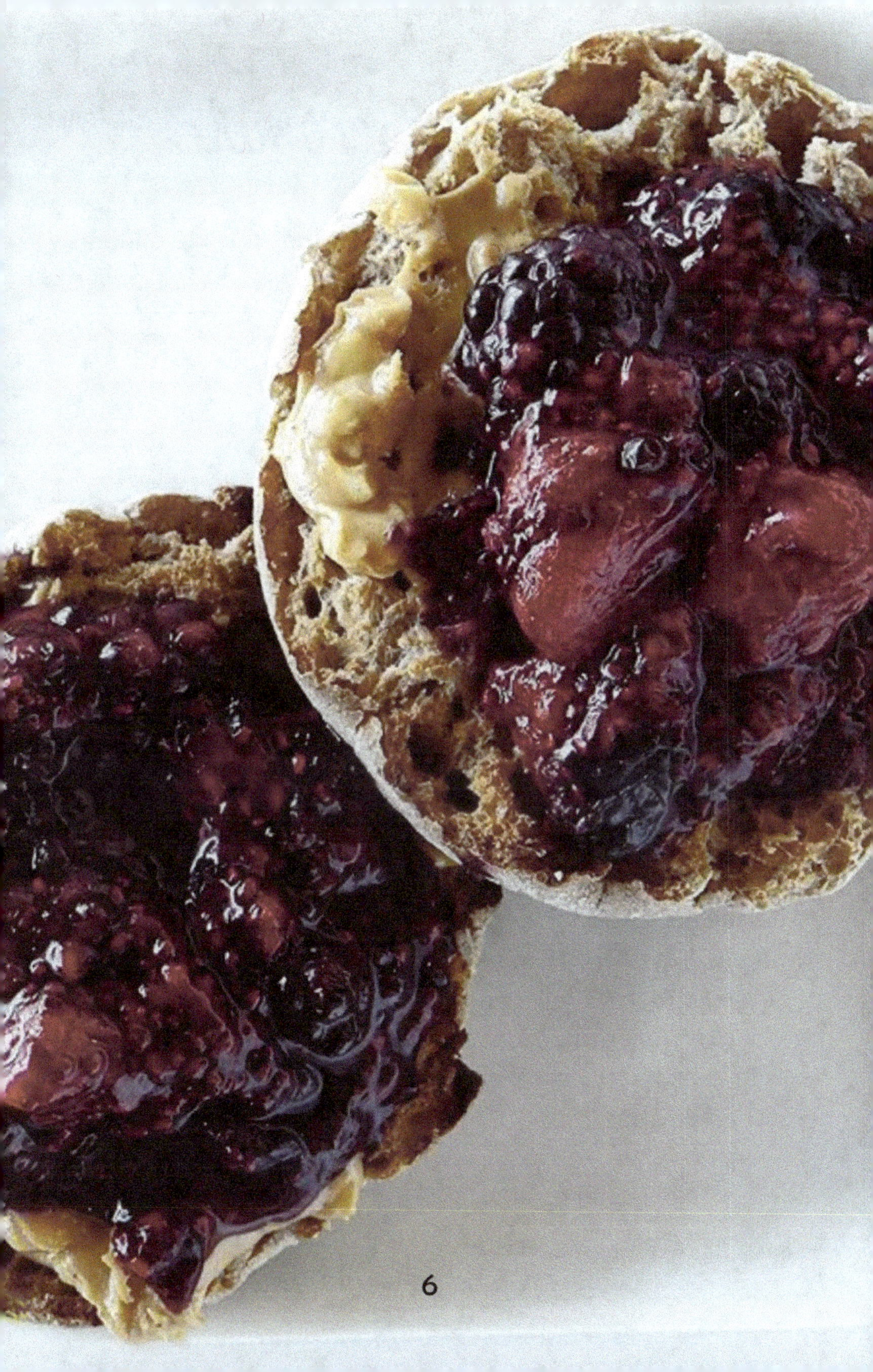

Spinach & Egg Scramble
With Raspberries

🍴 1 servings   🕐 10 minutes

INGREDIENTS

1 teaspoon canola oil

1 ½ cups baby spinach (1 1/2 ounces)

2 large eggs, lightly beaten

Pinch of kosher salt

Pinch of ground pepper

1 slice whole-grain bread, toasted

½ cup fresh raspberries

DIRECTIONS

1. Heat oil in a small nonstick skillet over medium-high heat. Add spinach and cook until wilted, stirring often, 1 to 2 minutes. Transfer the spinach to a plate. Wipe the pan clean, place over medium heat and add eggs. Cook, stirring once or twice to ensure even cooking, until just set, 1 to 2 minutes. Stir in the spinach, salt and pepper. Serve the scramble with toast and raspberries.

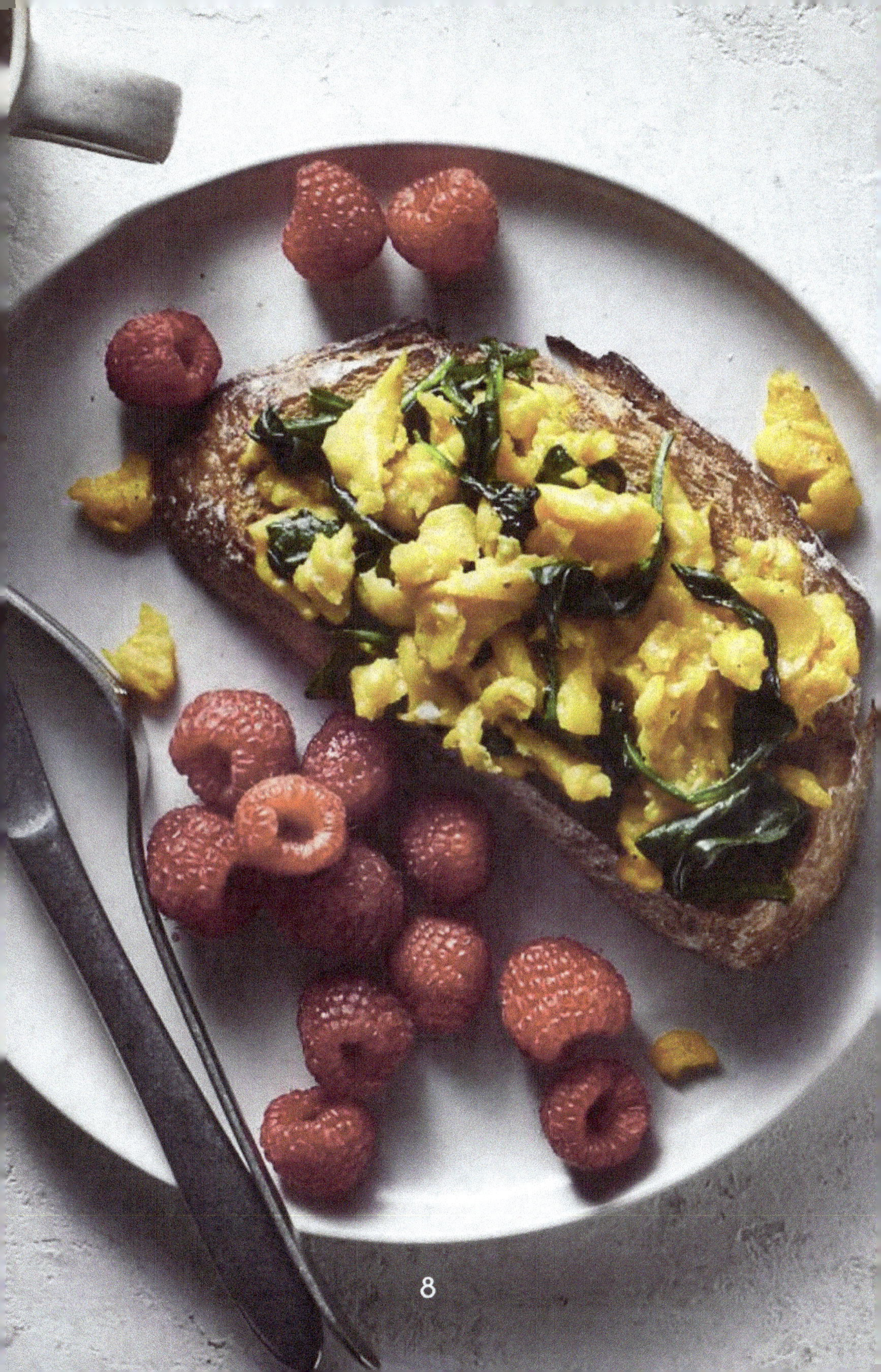

Muesli

With Raspberries

🍴 1 servings

🕐 5 minutes

INGREDIENTS

⅓ cup muesli

1 cup raspberries

¾ cup low-fat milk

DIRECTIONS

1. Top muesli with raspberries and serve with milk.

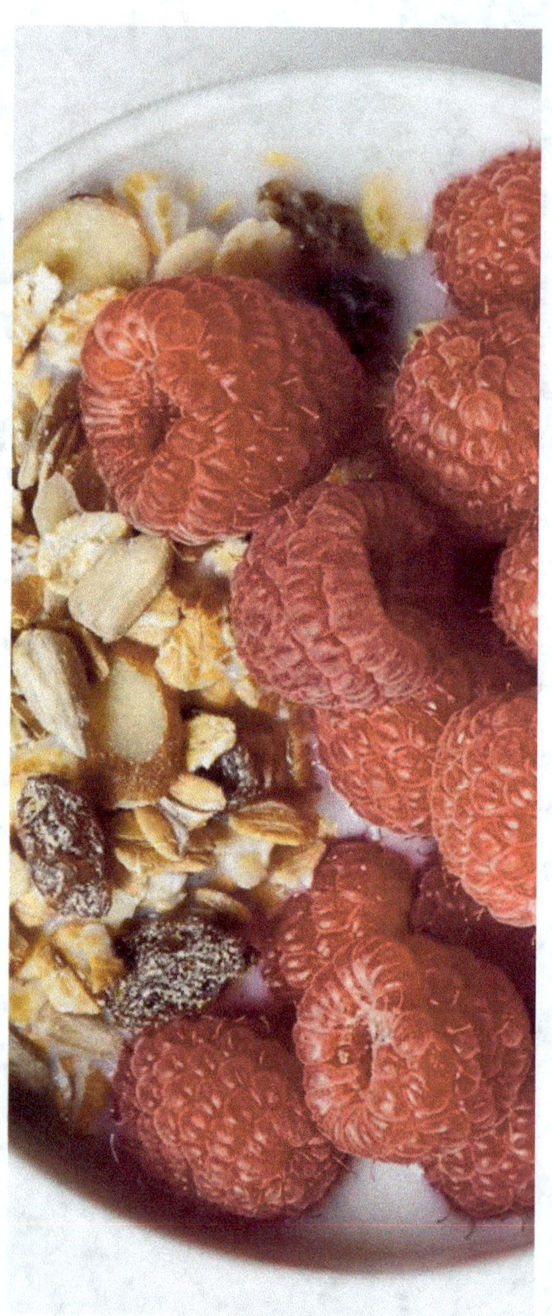

Breakfast Beans

with Microwave-Poached Egg

🍴 2 servings   🕐 15 minutes

INGREDIENTS

2 teaspoons canola oil

¼ cup chopped red bell pepper

2 chopped scallions, whites and greens separated

½ teaspoon ground cumin

¾ cup rinsed canned low-sodium black beans

½ cup cooked barley

½ cup low-sodium chicken broth or vegetable broth

⅛ teaspoon salt

⅛ teaspoon hot sauce

1 cup water, divided

1 teaspoon distilled white vinegar, divided

2 large eggs, divided

2 tablespoons shredded pepper Jack cheese

½ avocado, sliced

2 tablespoons coarsely chopped fresh cilantro

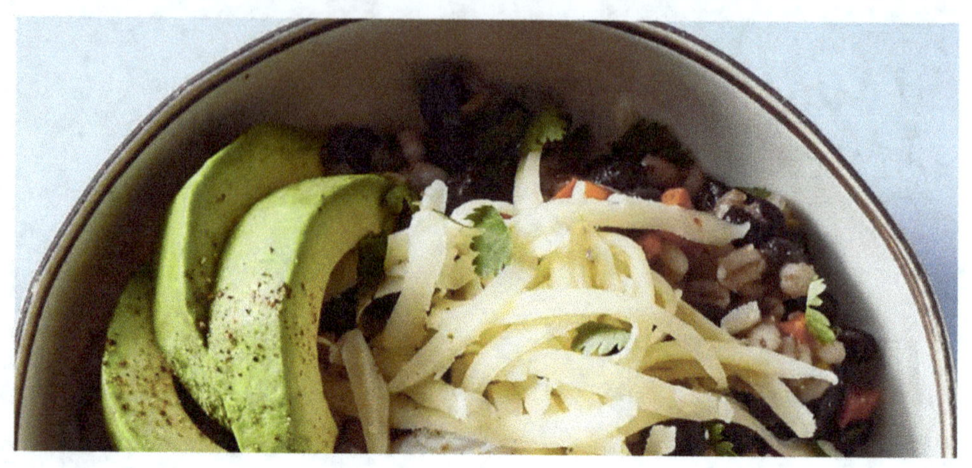

DIRECTIONS

1. Heat oil in a medium skillet over medium heat. Add bell pepper, scallion whites, and cumin; cook, stirring often, until softened, 1 to 2 minutes. Add beans, cooked barley, broth, and salt. Cook until most of the liquid is absorbed, 3 to 5 minutes. Stir in scallion greens and hot sauce. Divide between 2 bowls.

2. Place 1/2 cup water and 1/2 tsp. vinegar in a microwave-safe small bowl. Carefully crack 1 egg into the water so it is completely submerged. Cover with a microwave-safe plate and microwave on High until the egg white is firm and the yolk is still somewhat runny, about 1 minute. (If necessary, continue to microwave, checking every 10 seconds.) Remove the egg with a slotted spoon, pat dry and place atop the bean mixture in 1 bowl. Repeat with the remaining 1/2 cup water, 1/2 tsp. vinegar, and egg.

3. Top each bowl with 1 Tbsp. cheese and 1/4 avocado. Sprinkle with cilantro, if desired.

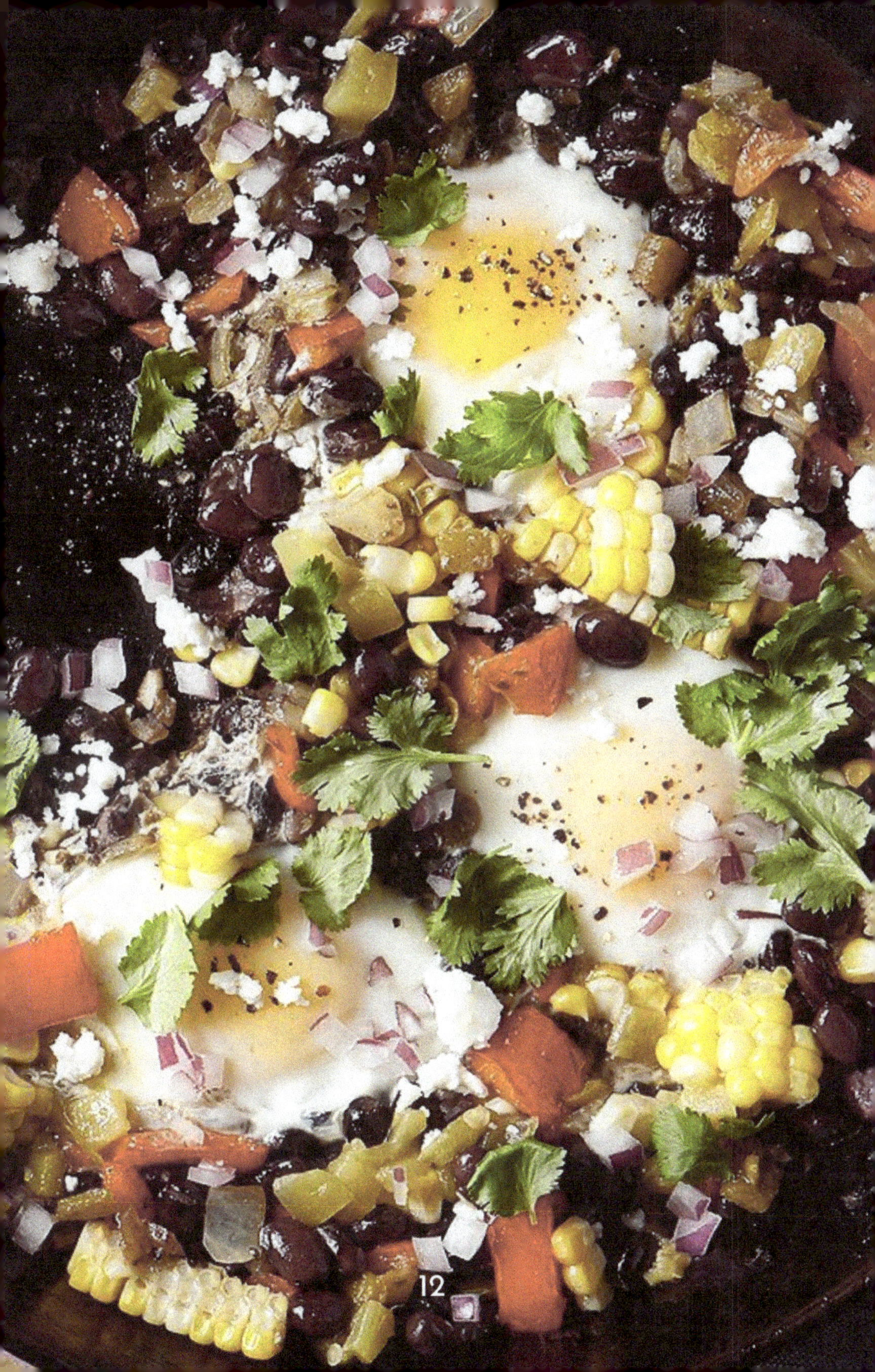

Egg Tartine

🍴 4 servings   🕐 10 minutes

INGREDIENTS

1 ½ teaspoons extra-virgin olive oil

4 slices whole-wheat bread, lightly toasted

1 garlic clove, halved

1 medium tomato or avocado, sliced

4 large eggs, fried or poached

2 tablespoons herbs or microgreens

4 teaspoons capers, rinsed

DIRECTIONS

1. Brush oil onto toast, then rub with garlic. Top with tomato (and/or avocado) and eggs. Sprinkle with herbs (or microgreens) and capers.

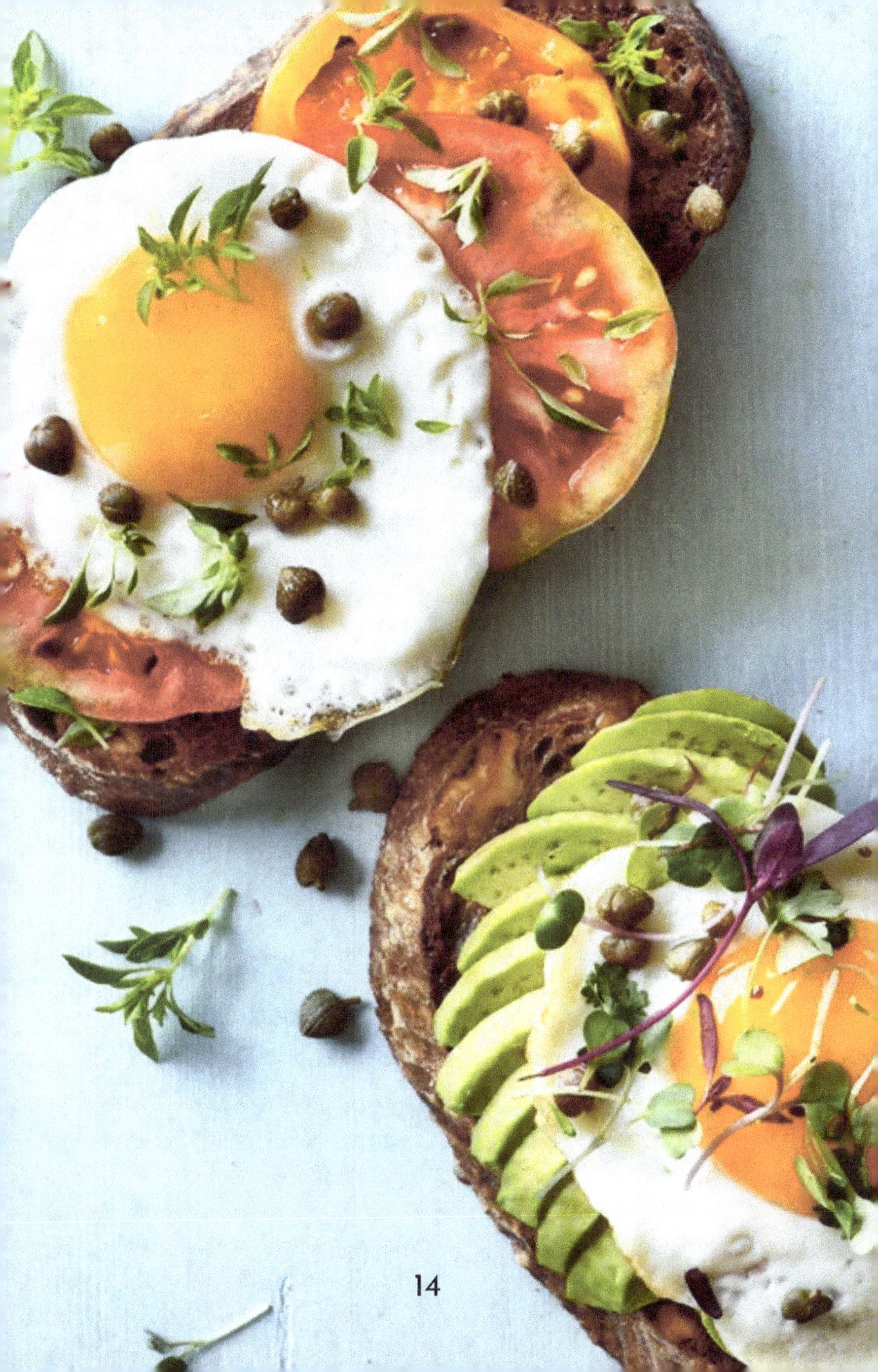

Pistachio & Peach Toast

1 servings　5 minutes

INGREDIENTS

1 tablespoon part-skim ricotta cheese

1 teaspoon honey, divided

⅛ teaspoon cinnamon

1 slice 100% whole-wheat bread, toasted

½ medium peach, sliced

1 tablespoon chopped pistachios

DIRECTIONS

1. Combine ricotta, ½ teaspoon honey and cinnamon in a small bowl.
2. Spread the ricotta mixture on toast and top with peach and pistachios. Drizzle with the remaining 1/2 teaspoon honey.

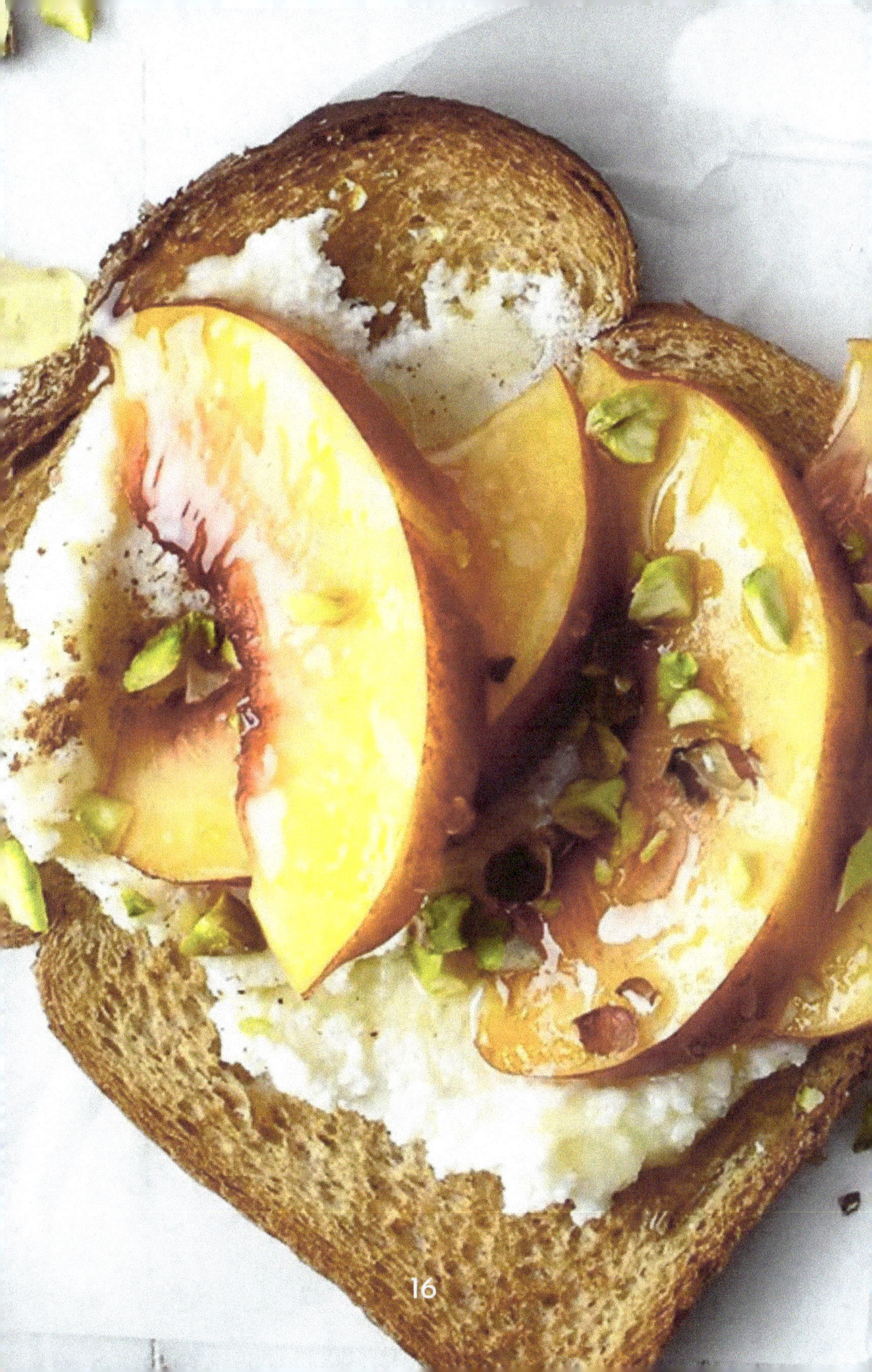

Baby Kale Breakfast Salad

with Smoked Trout & Avocado

🍴 1 servings   🕐 15 minutes

INGREDIENTS

1 teaspoon minced garlic

Pinch of salt

1 tablespoon extra-virgin olive oil

2 teaspoons red-wine vinegar

Pinch of pepper

3 cups lightly packed baby kale

¼ cup flaked smoked trout

¼ firm ripe avocado, sliced or diced

1 tablespoon finely chopped red onion

DIRECTIONS

1. Mash garlic and salt together with the side of a chef's knife to form a paste. Whisk the garlic paste, oil, vinegar and pepper together in a medium bowl. Add kale; toss to coat. Serve topped with trout, avocado and red onion.

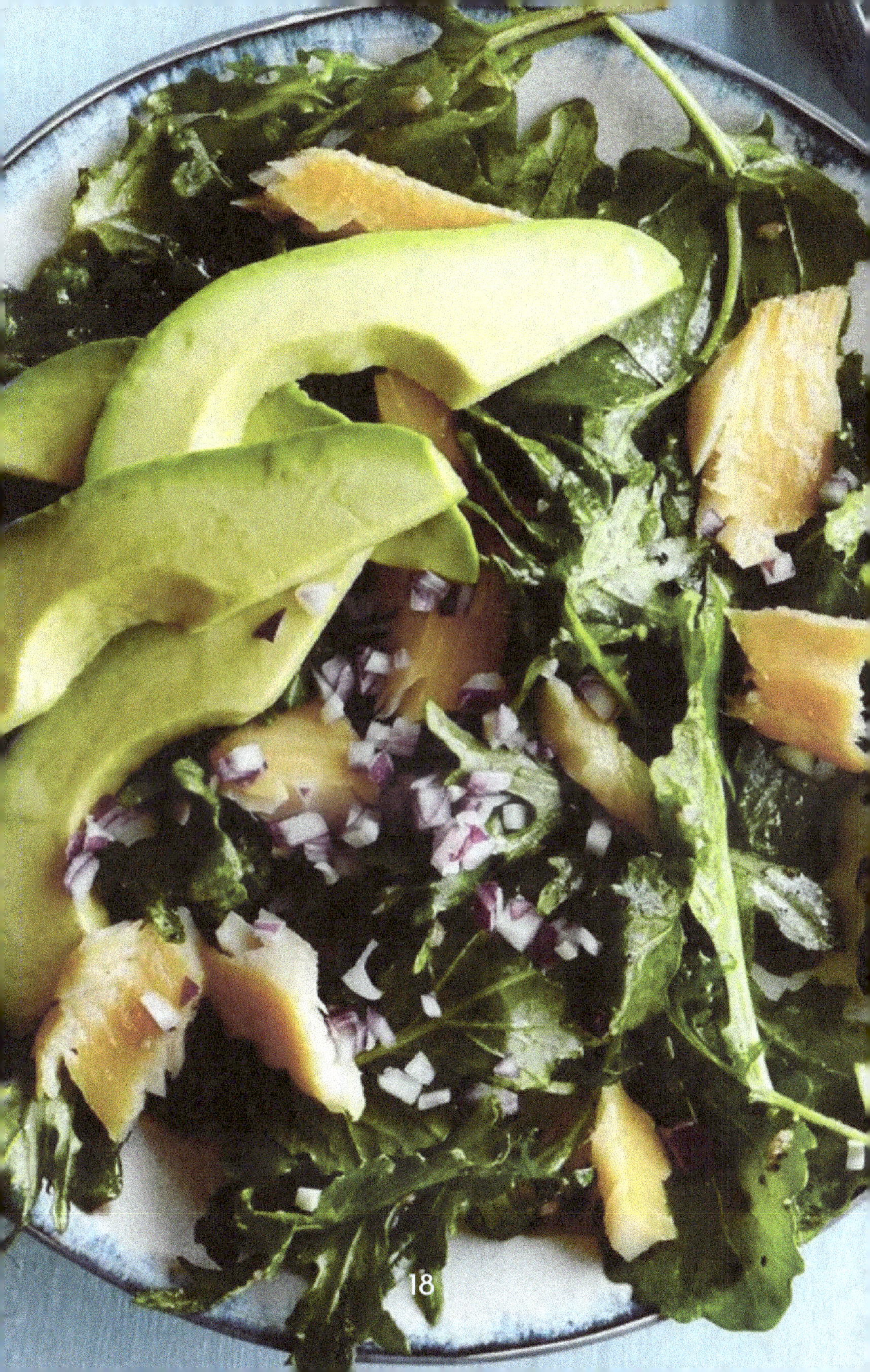

Lunch

Edamame & Veggie Rice Bowl

🍴 1 servings   🕐 5 minutes

INGREDIENTS

½ cup cooked brown rice

1 cup roasted vegetables

¼ cup edamame

¼ avocado, diced

2 tablespoons sliced scallions

2 tablespoons chopped fresh cilantro

2 tablespoons Citrus-Lime Vinaigrette

DIRECTIONS

1. Arrange rice, veggies, edamame and avocado in a 4-cup sealable container or bowl. Top with scallions and cilantro. Drizzle with vinaigrette just before serving.

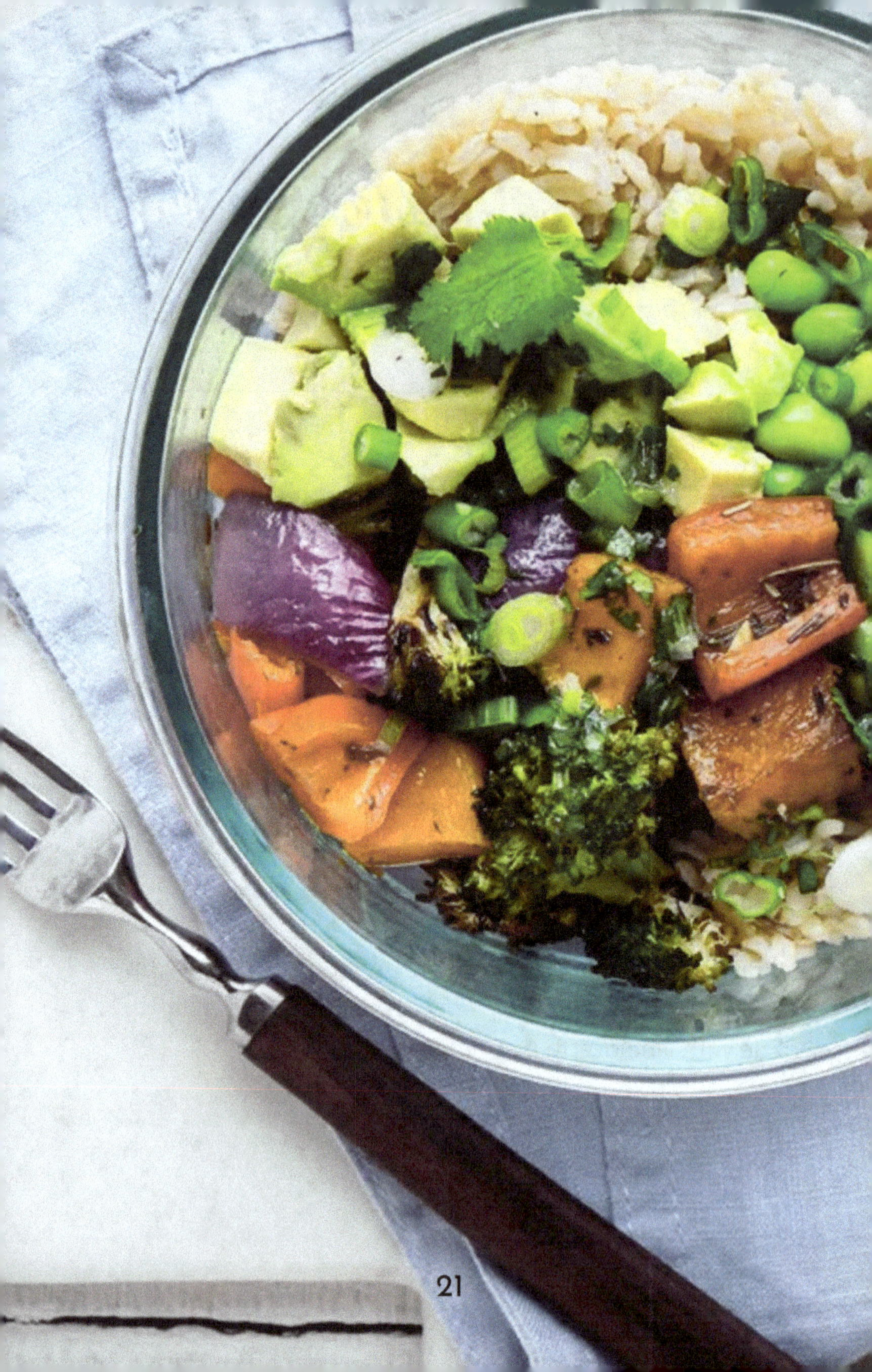

3-Ingredient Chicken Tabbouleh Bowls

🍴 2 servings   🕐 5 minutes

INGREDIENTS

1 (8 ounce) container prepared tabbouleh salad

½ cup hummus

6 ounces cooked chicken breast, sliced or shredded

DIRECTIONS

1. Divide tabbouleh salad between 2 shallow bowls. Top each with ¼ cup hummus and 3 ounces chicken.

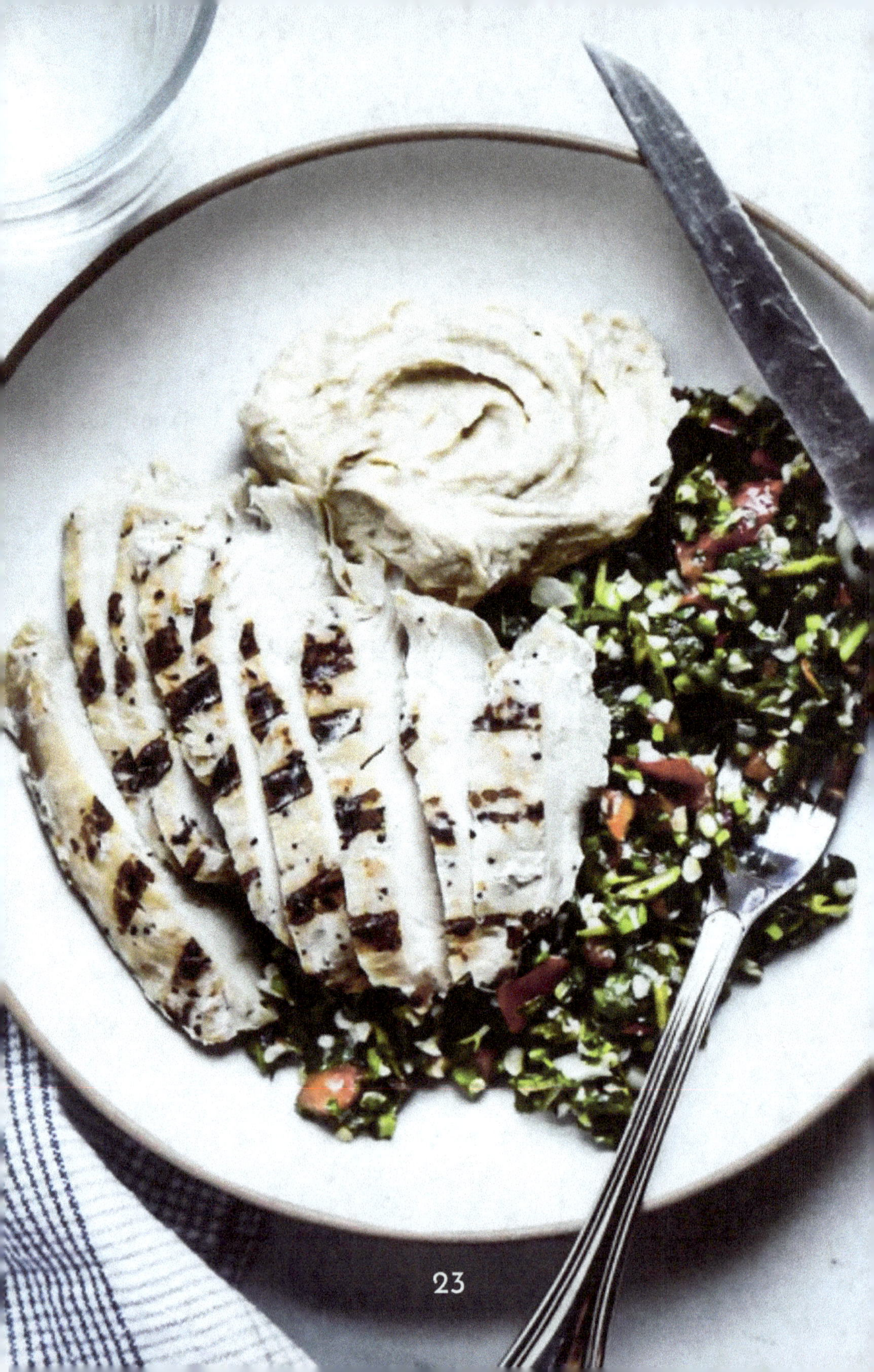

Smoked Salmon & Avocado Toasts

🍴 12 servings   🕐 15 minutes

INGREDIENTS

1 ripe avocado, pitted

2 teaspoons lemon juice

1 teaspoon minced fresh tarragon

24 toasted cocktail-size slices pumpernickel bread or melba toasts

2 ounces smoked salmon, cut into 24 pieces

1 teaspoon coarse Maldon sea salt

Fresh tarragon sprigs, capers, sliced cornichons or olives, poppy or sesame seeds, lemon zest and/or red onion for garnish

DIRECTIONS

1. Mash avocado with lemon juice and tarragon in a bowl. Spread about 1 teaspoon of the mixture on each piece of bread (or toast). Top with salmon and sprinkle with salt. Garnish as desired.

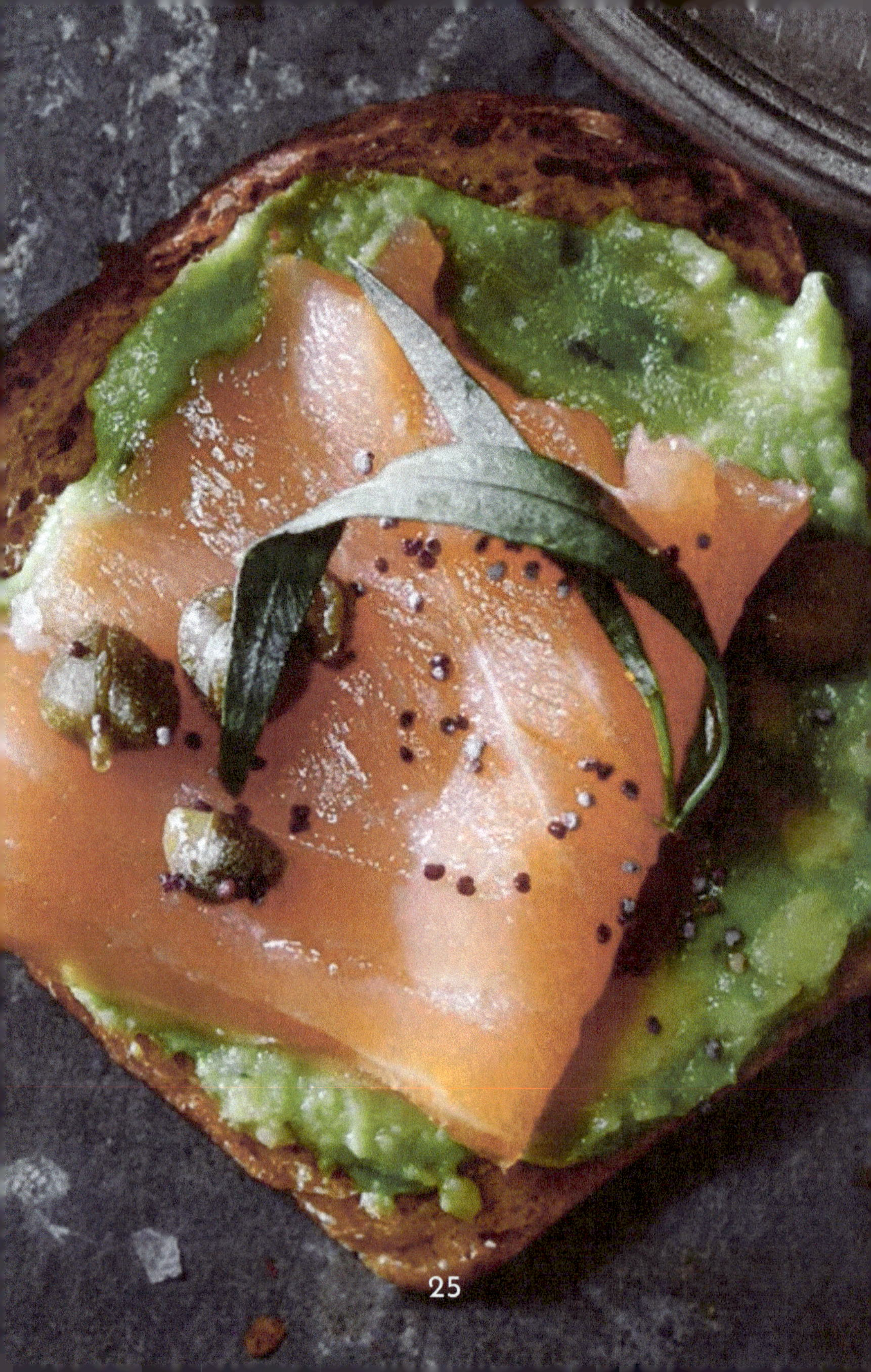

Kale Turkey Wraps

🍴 1 servings   🕐 10 minutes

INGREDIENTS

1 tablespoon cranberry sauce

1 teaspoon Dijon mustard

3 medium lacinato kale leaves

3 slices deli turkey (about 3 ounces)

6 thin red onion slices

1 firm ripe pear, cut into 9 slices

DIRECTIONS

1. Mix cranberry sauce and mustard in a small bowl. Spread on kale leaves. Top each leaf with a slice of turkey, 2 slices red onion and 3 slices pear. Roll each leaf into a wrap. Cut each wrap in half, if desired.

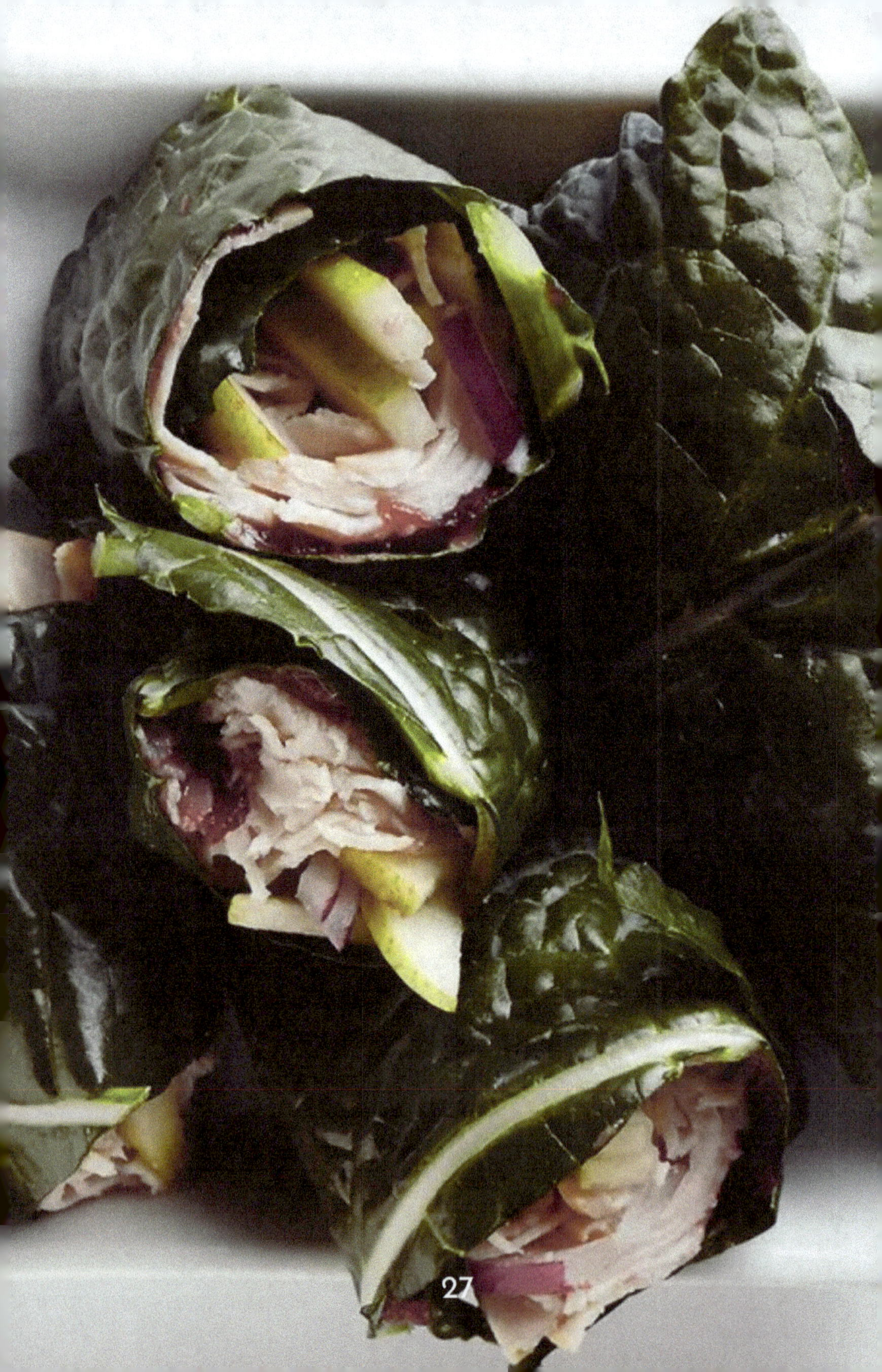

Chopped Veggie Grain Bowls

with Turmeric Dressing

🍴 4 servings   🕐 10 minutes

INGREDIENTS

2 (8 ounce) packages cooked quinoa

1 (16 ounce) container chopped veggie mix

1 (15.5 ounce) can chickpeas, rinsed

1/2 cup creamy turmeric salad dressing

DIRECTIONS

1. Prepare quinoa according to package directions. Transfer to a shallow bowl to cool completely before assembling bowls.
2. Divide veggie mix among 4 single-serving lidded containers. Top each with one-fourth of the quinoa and one-fourth of the chickpeas. Seal the containers and refrigerate for up to 4 days.
3. Transfer 2 tablespoons salad dressing into each of 4 small lidded containers and refrigerate for up to 4 days.
4. Toss each bowl with dressing just before serving.

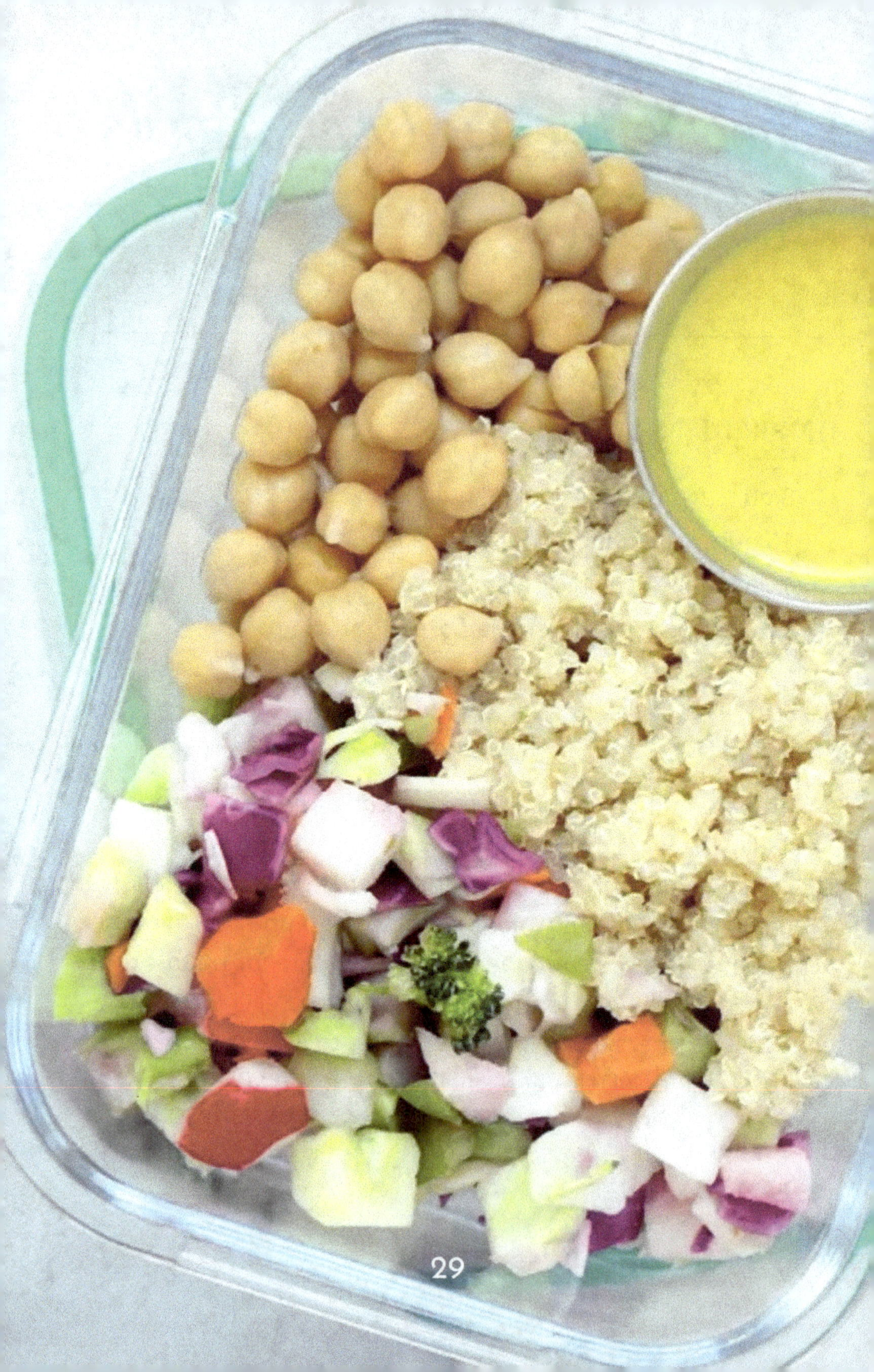

Couscous & Chickpea Salad

🍴 1 servings   🕐 5 minutes

INGREDIENTS

1 cup finely chopped kale

¾ cup cooked whole-wheat couscous

⅔ cup rinsed canned chickpeas

4 tablespoons Basil Vinaigrette

DIRECTIONS

1. Combine kale, couscous, chickpeas and dressing in a medium bowl. Serve immediately or refrigerate in a sealable container for up to 4 days.

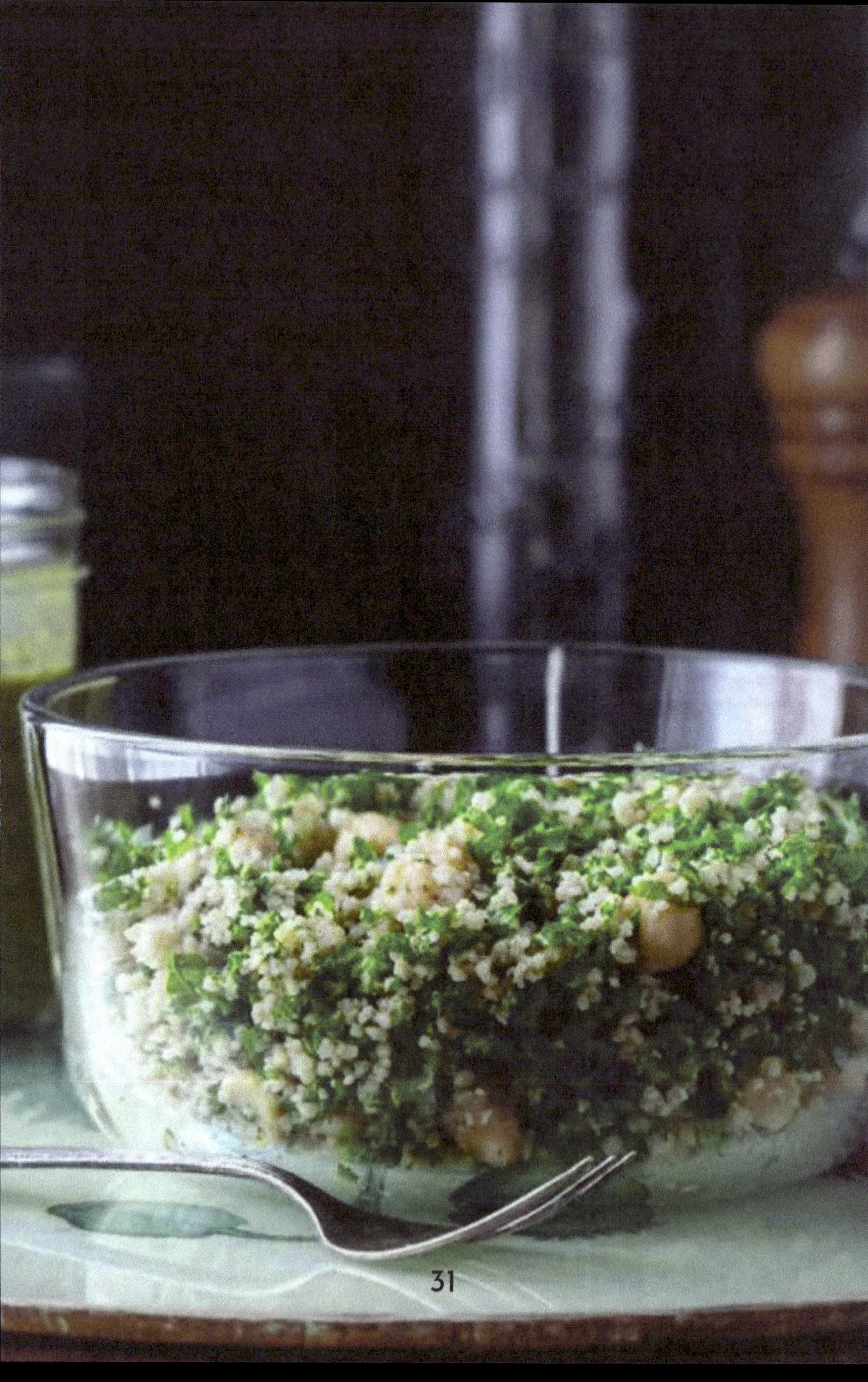

Kale Salad

With Balsamic & Parmesan

🍴 6 servings   🕐 15 minutes

INGREDIENTS

3 tablespoons extra-virgin olive oil

3 tablespoons balsamic vinegar

1 large clove garlic, grated

¼ teaspoon salt

¼ teaspoon ground pepper

10 cups roughly chopped kale

⅓ cup grated Parmesan cheese

¼ cup toasted pine nuts

DIRECTIONS

1. Whisk oil, vinegar, garlic, salt and pepper in a large bowl; add kale. With clean hands, firmly massage the kale to work in the dressing. Stop when the greens are softened and reduced in volume. Stir in Parmesan and pine nuts.

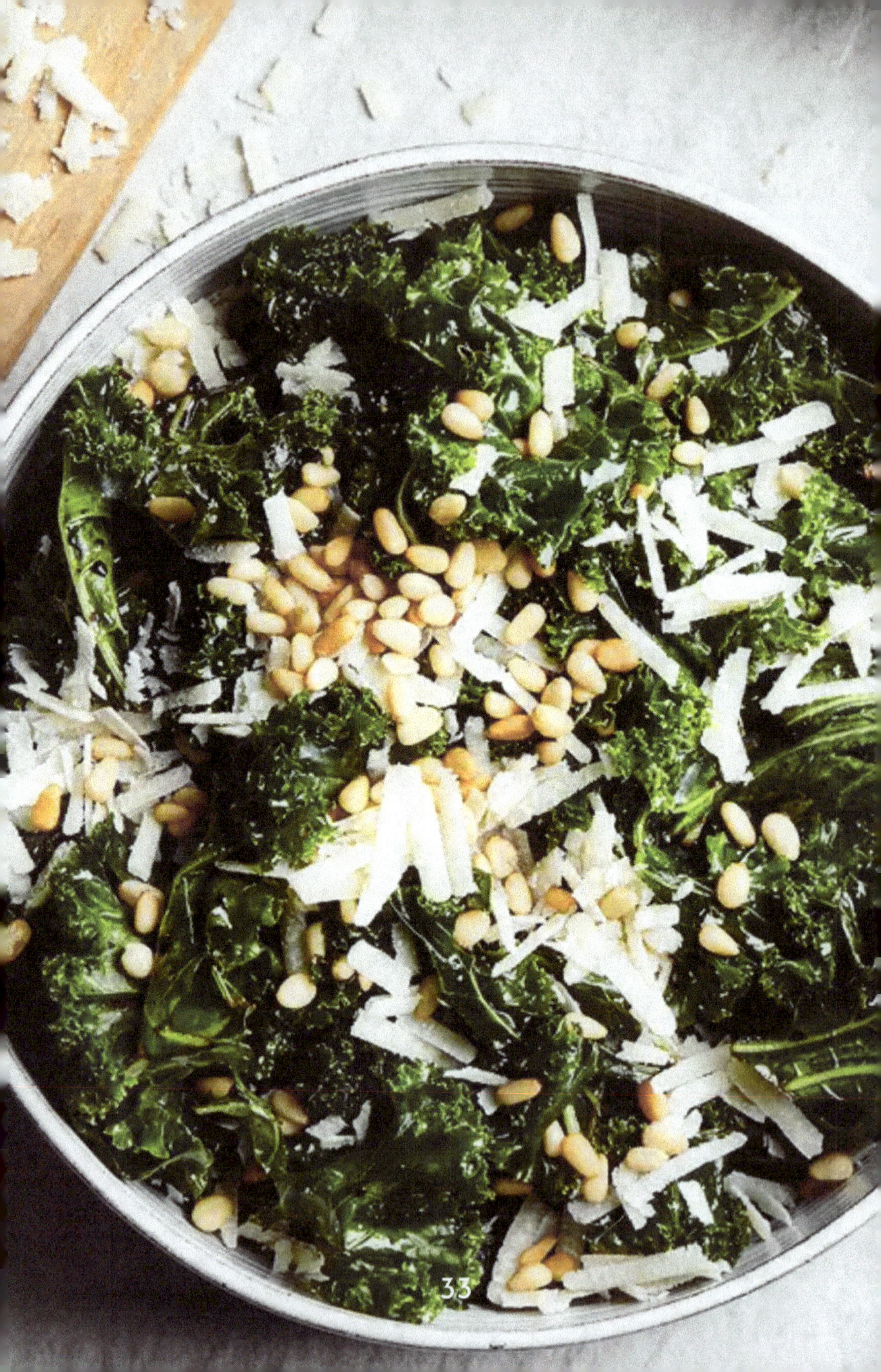

Honey Walnut Shrimp

🍴 4 servings   🕐 15 minutes

INGREDIENTS

2 tablespoons water

2 tablespoons light brown sugar

½ cup walnuts, coarsely chopped

1 pound jumbo peeled, deveined raw shrimp

1 tablespoon honey

2 tablespoons extra-virgin olive oil, divided

2 ½ tablespoons mayonnaise

1 tablespoon lemon juice

½ teaspoon ground pepper

¼ teaspoon salt

½ cup sliced scallions

2 cups hot cooked brown rice or white rice (Optional)

DIRECTIONS

1. Bring water and brown sugar to a simmer in a large nonstick skillet over medium heat; cook until the sugar is completely dissolved, about 2 minutes. Stir in walnuts; cook, stirring often, until the sugar is golden and caramelized, about 2 minutes. Spread the walnuts evenly on a parchment paper-lined plate. Wipe out the pan.

2. Stir shrimp, honey and 1 tablespoon oil together in a bowl. Return the skillet to medium-high heat. Add the shrimp mixture; cook, stirring occasionally, until the shrimp are well browned and cooked through, about 4 minutes. Remove from heat. Combine mayonnaise, lemon juice, pepper, salt and the remaining 1 tablespoon oil in a small bowl; add to the shrimp mixture in the pan, stirring to coat. Sprinkle with the caramelized walnuts and scallions. If desired, serve with rice.

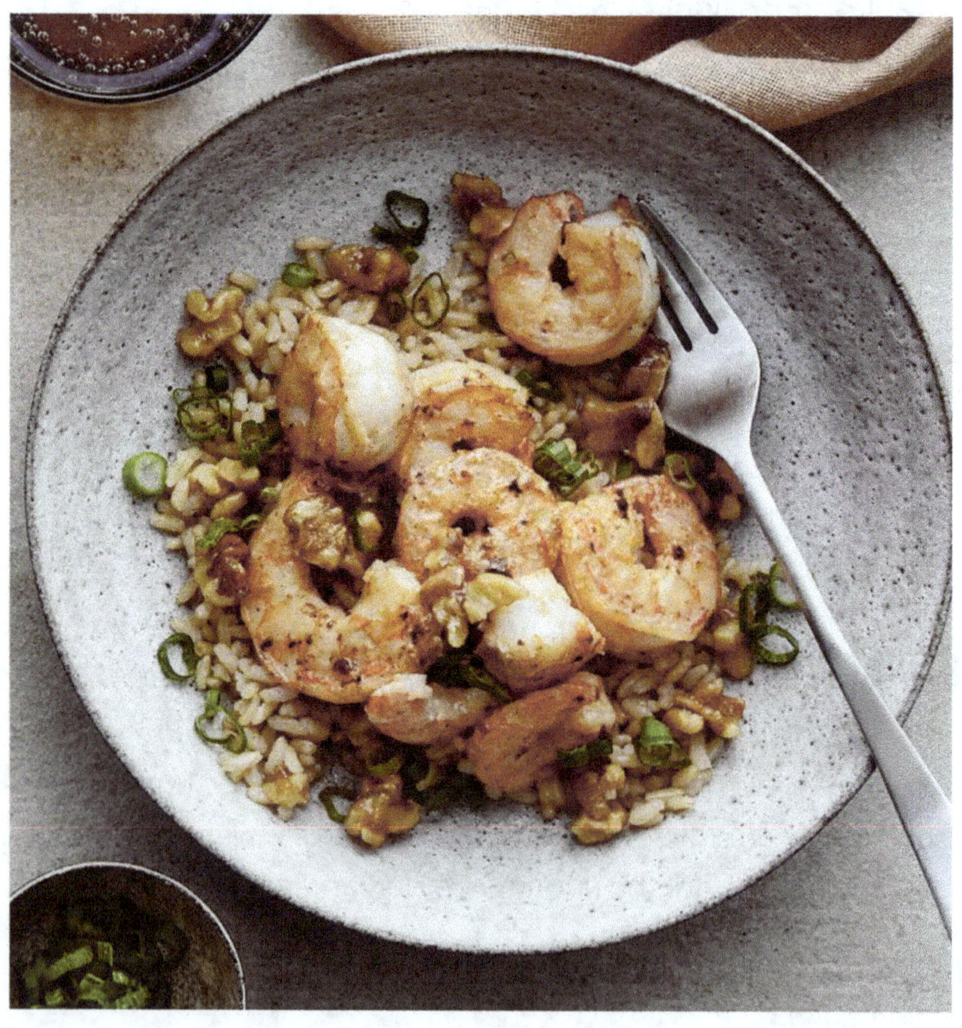

Tuna Salad with Egg

🍴 4 servings   🕐 15 minutes

INGREDIENTS

¾ cup finely chopped celery

½ cup coarsely chopped arugula

¼ cup mayonnaise

¼ cup thinly sliced scallions, white and light green parts only

¼ cup whole-milk plain Greek yogurt

1 teaspoon grated lemon zest

2 tablespoons lemon juice

1 ½ tablespoons capers, rinsed

½ teaspoon dried tarragon, rubbed

2 (5 ounce) cans solid white tuna in water, drained

2 hard-boiled eggs, chopped

DIRECTIONS

1. Stir celery, arugula, mayonnaise, scallions, yogurt, lemon zest, lemon juice, capers and tarragon together in a medium bowl until well combined. Gently fold in tuna and eggs. Serve over salad greens or on sandwich bread, if desired.

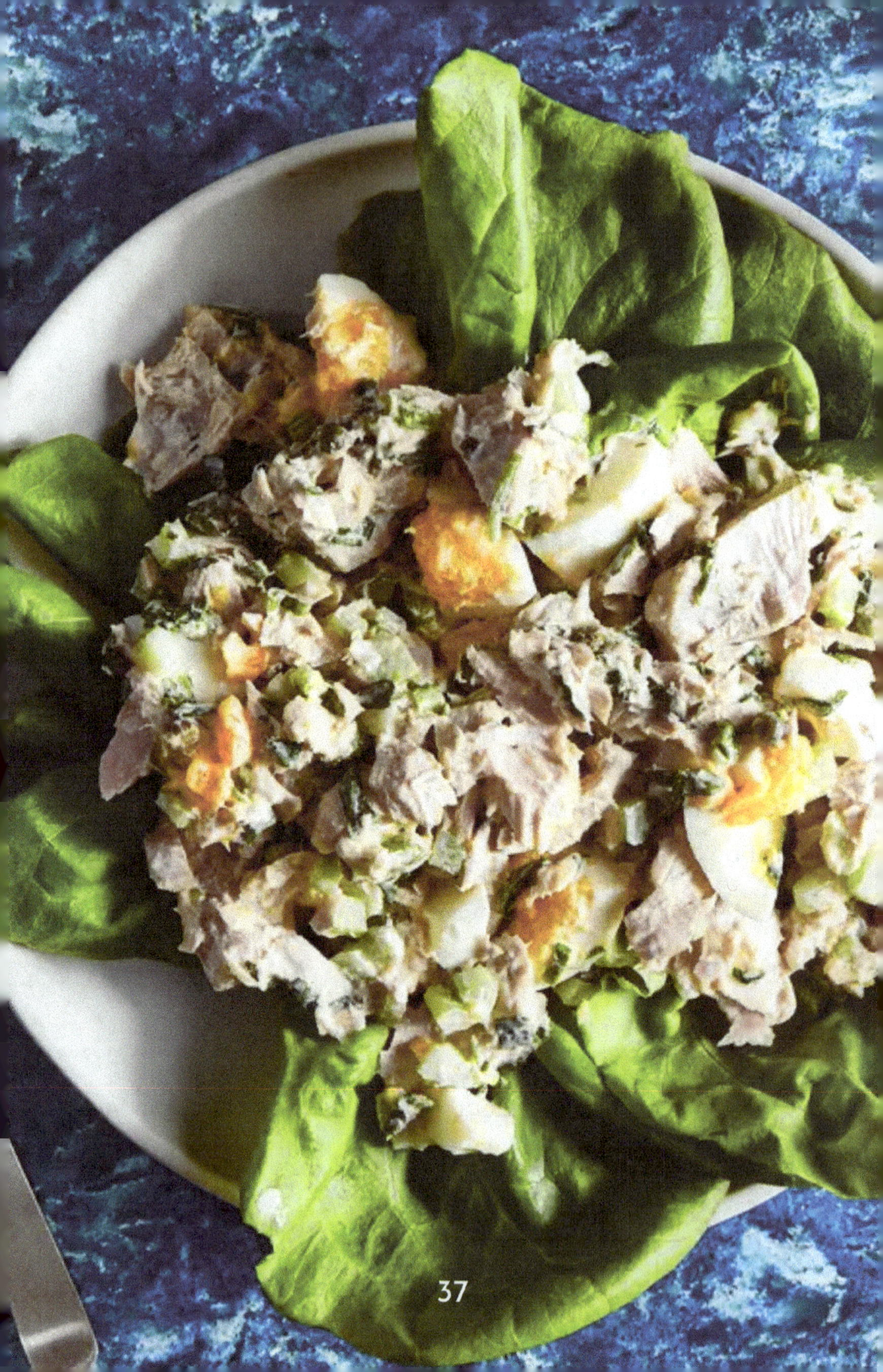

Dinner

Mushroom & Tofu Stir-Fry

🍴 4 servings   🕐 15 minutes

INGREDIENTS

4 tablespoons peanut oil or canola oil, divided

1 pound mixed mushrooms, sliced

1 medium red bell pepper, diced

1 bunch scallions, trimmed and cut into 2-inch pieces

1 tablespoon grated fresh ginger

1 large clove garlic, grated

1 (8 ounce) container baked tofu or smoked tofu, diced

3 tablespoons oyster sauce or vegetarian oyster sauce

DIRECTIONS

1. Heat 2 tablespoons oil in a large flat-bottom wok or cast-iron skillet over high heat. Add mushrooms and bell pepper; cook, stirring occasionally, until soft, about 4 minutes. Stir in scallions, ginger and garlic; cook for 30 seconds more. Transfer the vegetables to a bowl.

2. Add the remaining 2 tablespoons oil and tofu to the pan. Cook, turning once, until browned, 3 to 4 minutes. Stir in the vegetables and oyster sauce. Cook, stirring, until hot, about 1 minute.

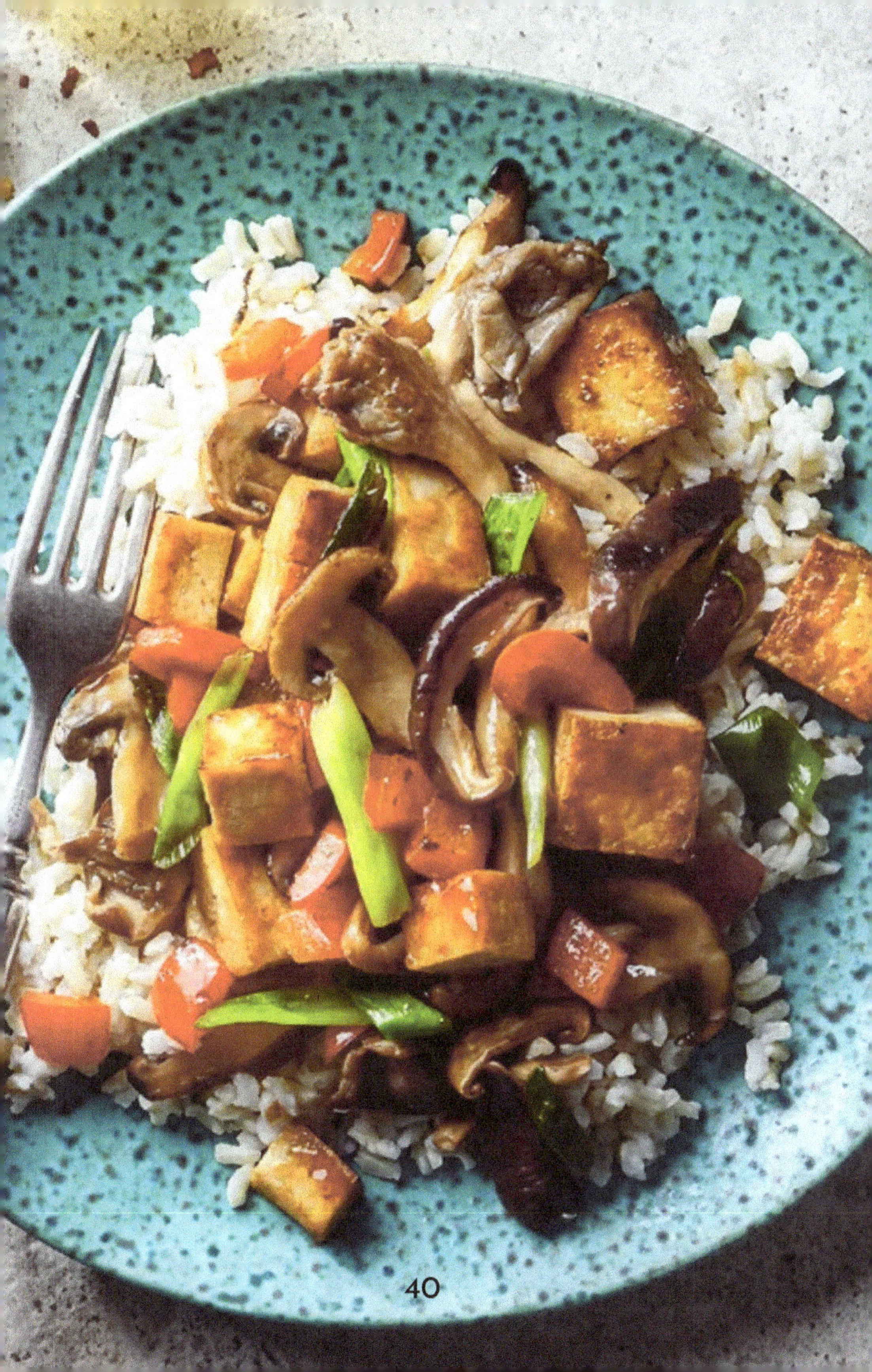

Pan-Seared Steak

With Crispy Herbs & Escarole

🍴 4 servings　　🕐 20 minutes

INGREDIENTS

1 pound sirloin steak, about 1/2 inch thick

½ teaspoon salt, divided

½ teaspoon ground pepper, divided

2 tablespoons grapeseed oil or canola oil

4 cloves garlic, crushed

5 sprigs fresh thyme

3 sprigs fresh sage

1 sprig fresh rosemary

16 cups chopped escarole (about 1 pound)

DIRECTIONS

1. Sprinkle steak with 1/4 teaspoon each salt and pepper. Heat a large cast-iron skillet over medium-high heat. Add the steak and cook until charred on one side, about 3 minutes. Turn the steak over and add oil, garlic, thyme, sage and rosemary. Cook, stirring the herbs occasionally, until an instant-read thermometer inserted in the thickest part of the steak reaches 125 degrees F for medium-rare, 3 to 4 minutes.

2. Transfer the steak to a plate and top with the garlic and herbs. Tent with foil.

3. Add escarole and the remaining 1/4 teaspoon each salt and pepper to the pan. Cook, stirring often, until the escarole starts to wilt, about 2 minutes. Thinly slice the steak and serve with the escarole and crispy herbs.

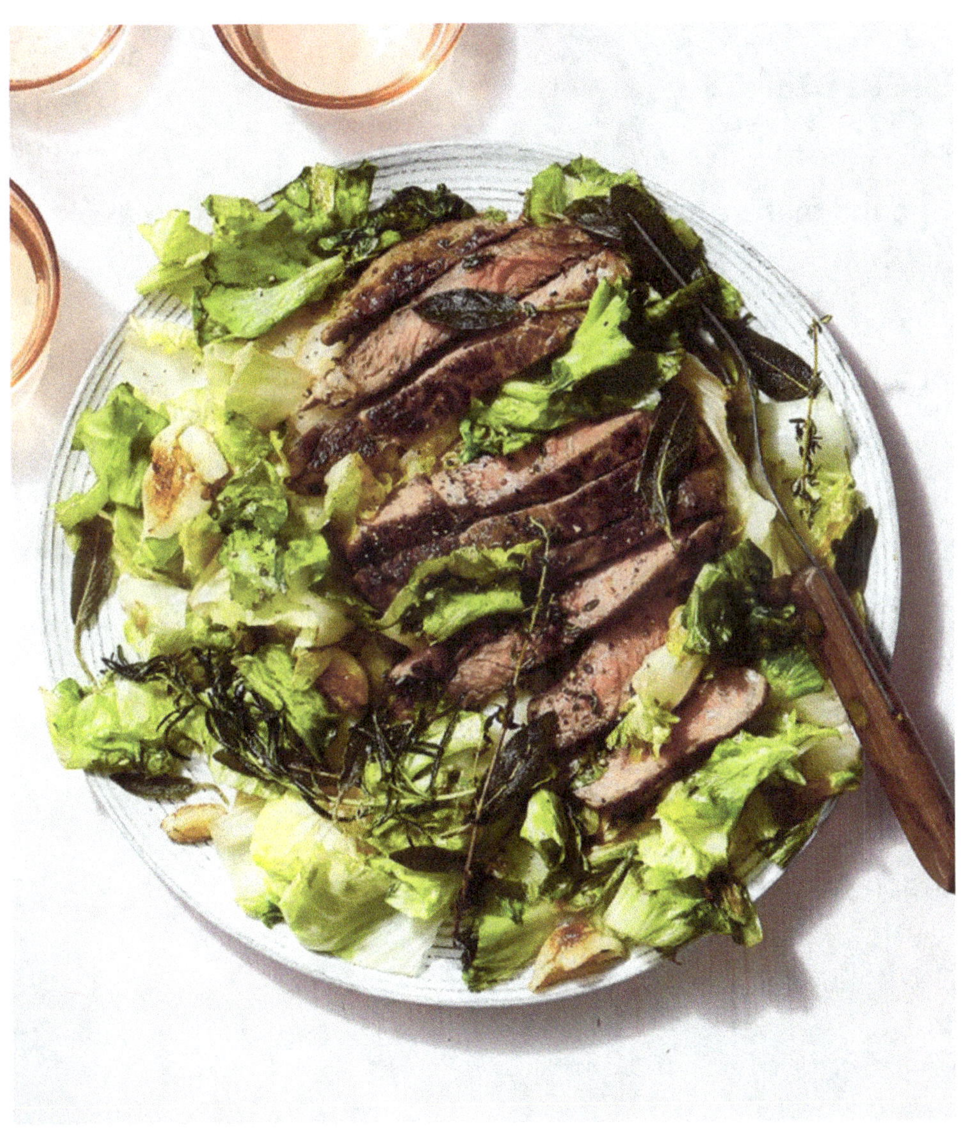

Seared Scallops

With White Bean Ragu & Charred Lemon

🍴 4 servings   🕐 25 minutes

INGREDIENTS

3 teaspoons extra-virgin olive oil, divided

1 pound mature spinach or white chard, trimmed and thinly sliced

2 cloves garlic, minced

1 tablespoon capers, rinsed and chopped

½ teaspoon ground pepper, divided

1 (15 ounce) can no-salt-added cannellini beans, drained and rinsed

1 cup low-sodium chicken broth

⅓ cup dry white wine

1 tablespoon butter

1 pound dry sea scallops, tough side muscle removed

1 lemon, halved

2 tablespoons chopped fresh parsley

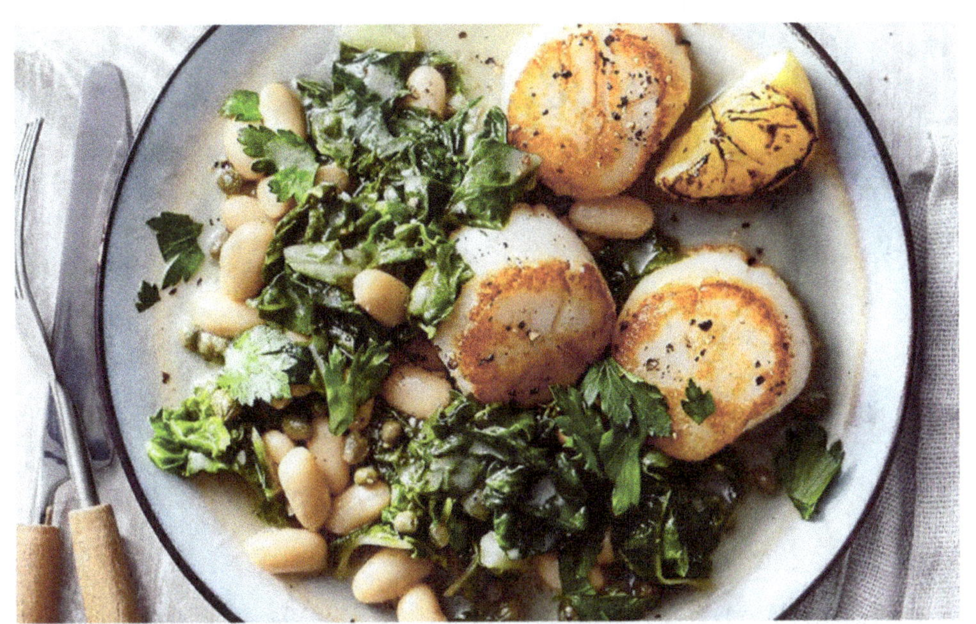

DIRECTIONS

1. Heat 2 teaspoons oil in a large skillet over medium-high heat. Add greens and cook, stirring often, until wilted, about 4 minutes. Stir in garlic, capers and 1/4 teaspoon pepper; cook, stirring occasionally, until fragrant, about 30 seconds. Add beans, broth and wine and bring to a simmer. Reduce heat to maintain a low simmer, cover and cook for 5 minutes. Remove from heat and stir in butter. Cover to keep warm.

2. Meanwhile, sprinkle scallops with the remaining 1/4 teaspoon pepper. Heat the remaining 1 teaspoon oil in a large nonstick skillet over medium-high heat. Add the scallops and cook until browned on both sides, about 4 minutes total. Transfer to a clean plate. Add lemon halves to the pan, cut-side down, and cook until charred, about 2 minutes. Cut into wedges. Sprinkle the scallops and the bean ragu with parsley and serve with the lemon wedges.

Roasted Vegetable & Black Bean Tacos

🍴 2 servings   🕐 15 minutes

INGREDIENTS

1 cup roasted root vegetables

½ cup cooked or canned black beans, rinsed

2 teaspoons extra-virgin olive oil

1 teaspoon ground cumin

1 teaspoon chili powder

½ teaspoon ground coriander

¼ teaspoon kosher salt

¼ teaspoon ground pepper

4 corn tortillas, lightly toasted or warmed

½ avocado, cut into 8 slices

1 lime, cut into wedges

Chopped fresh cilantro & salsa for garnish

DIRECTIONS

1. Combine roasted root vegetables, beans, oil, cumin, chili powder, coriander, salt and pepper in a saucepan. Cover and cook over medium-low heat until heated through, 6 to 8 minutes.

2.Divide the mixture among the tortillas. Top with avocado. Serve with lime wedges. Garnish with cilantro and/or salsa, if desired.

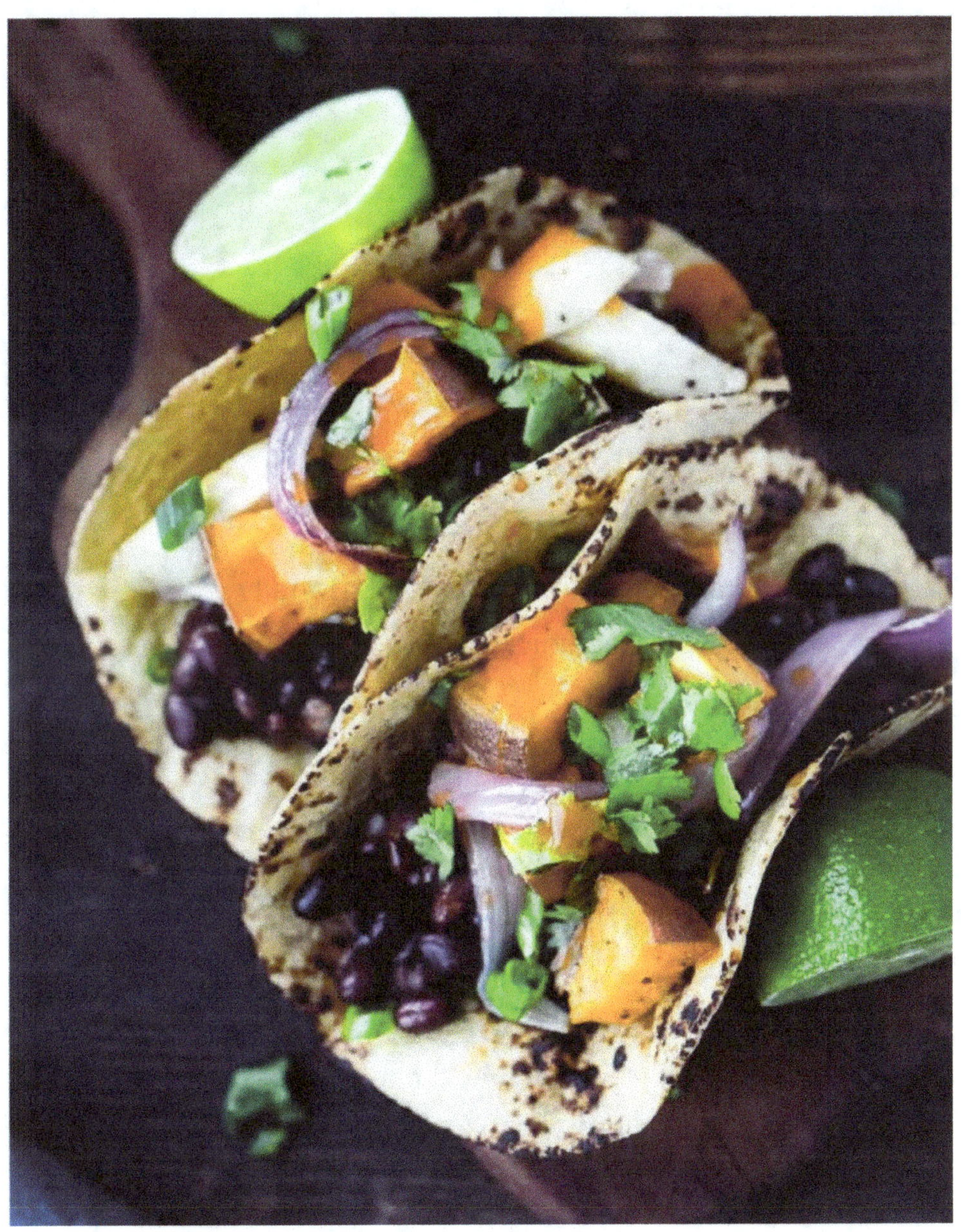

Crunchy Chicken & Mango Salad

🍴 12 servings   🕐 15 minutes

INGREDIENTS

⅓ cup orange juice

3 tablespoons rice vinegar

3 tablespoons less-sodium soy sauce

1 tablespoon toasted sesame oil

2 teaspoons sambal oelek (Optional)

6 cups thinly sliced napa cabbage

2 cups sugar snap peas, thinly sliced diagonally

2 cups shredded cooked chicken breast

1 medium mango, sliced

½ cup coarsely chopped fresh mint

¼ cup sliced scallions

2 tablespoons toasted sesame seeds

DIRECTIONS

1. Whisk juice, vinegar, soy sauce, sesame oil and sambal oelek (if using) in a large bowl. Add cabbage, peas, chicken, mango, mint and scallions; toss gently to coat. Serve the salad sprinkled with sesame seeds.

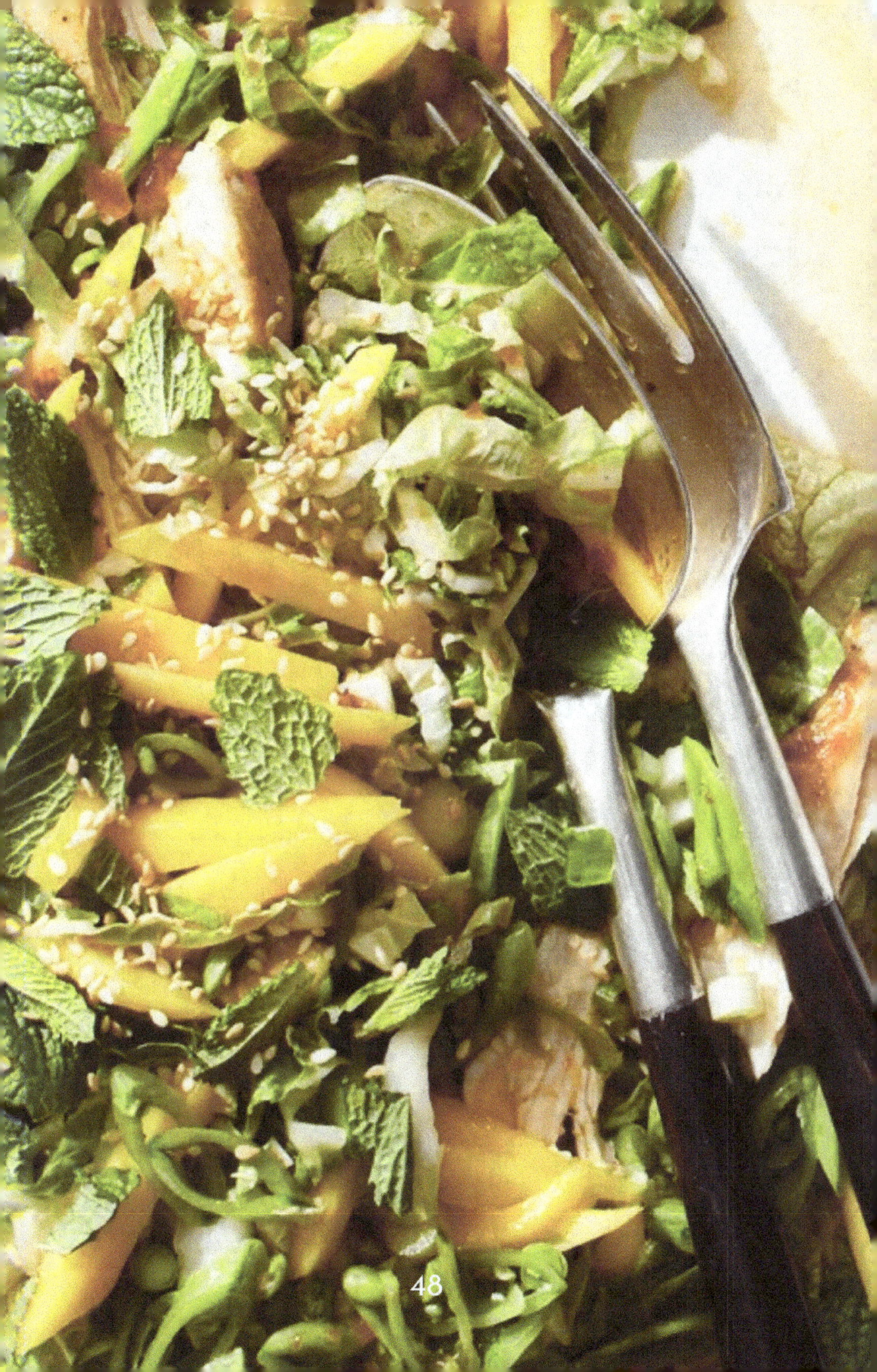

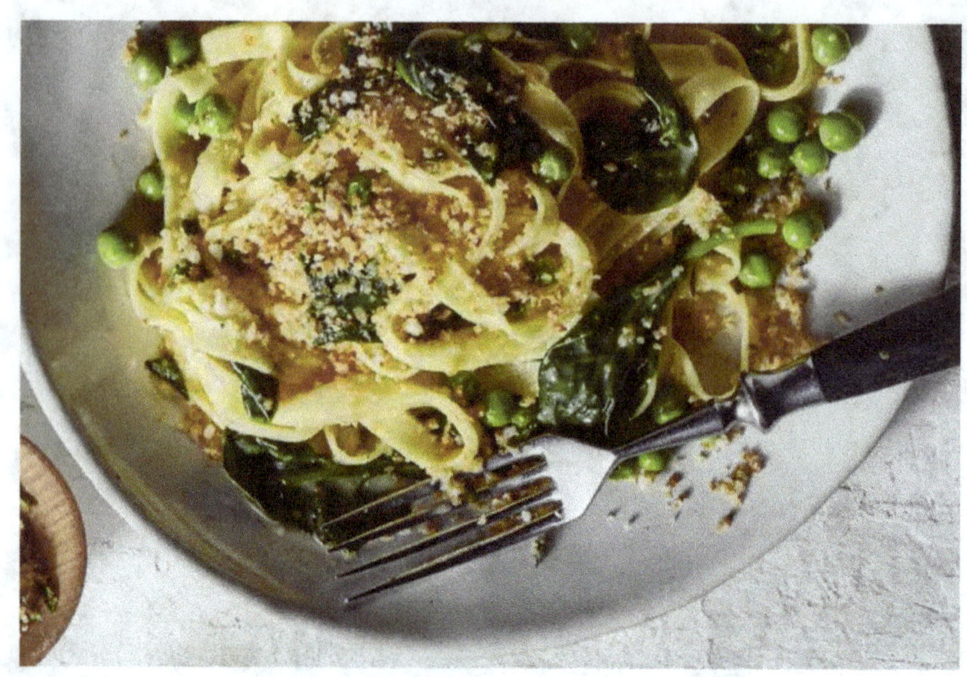

Pea & Spinach Carbonara

🍴 4 servings   🕐 20 minutes

INGREDIENTS

1 ½ tablespoons extra-virgin olive oil

½ cup panko breadcrumbs, preferably whole-wheat

1 small clove garlic, minced

8 tablespoons grated Parmesan cheese, divided

3 tablespoons finely chopped fresh parsley

3 large egg yolks

1 large egg
½ teaspoon ground pepper
¼ teaspoon salt
1 (9 ounce) package fresh tagliatelle or linguine
8 cups baby spinach
1 cup peas (fresh or frozen)

DIRECTIONS

1. Put 10 cups of water in a large pot and bring to a boil over high heat.
2. Meanwhile, heat oil in a large skillet over medium-high heat. Add breadcrumbs and garlic; cook, stirring frequently, until toasted, about 2 minutes. Transfer to a small bowl and stir in 2 tablespoons Parmesan and parsley. Set aside.
3. Whisk the remaining 6 tablespoons Parmesan, egg yolks, egg, pepper and salt in a medium bowl.
4. Cook pasta in the boiling water, stirring occasionally, for 1 minute. Add spinach and peas and cook until the pasta is tender, about 1 minute more. Reserve 1/4 cup of the cooking water. Drain and place in a large bowl.
5. Slowly whisk the reserved cooking water into the egg mixture. Gradually add the mixture to the pasta, tossing with tongs to combine. Serve topped with the reserved breadcrumb mixture.

Stuffed Potatoes
With Salsa & Beans

🍴 4 servings   🕐 25 minutes

INGREDIENTS

4 medium russet potatoes

½ cup fresh salsa

1 ripe avocado, sliced

1 (15 ounce) can pinto beans, rinsed, warmed and lightly mashed

4 teaspoons chopped pickled jalapeños

DIRECTIONS

1. Pierce potatoes all over with a fork. Microwave on Medium, turning once or twice, until soft, about 20 minutes. (Alternatively, bake potatoes at 425 degrees F until tender, 45 minutes to 1 hour.) Transfer to a clean cutting board and let cool slightly.
2. Holding them with a kitchen towel to protect your hands, make a lengthwise cut to open the potato, but don't cut all the way through. Pinch the ends to expose the flesh.
3. Top each potato with some salsa, avocado, beans and jalapeños. Serve warm.

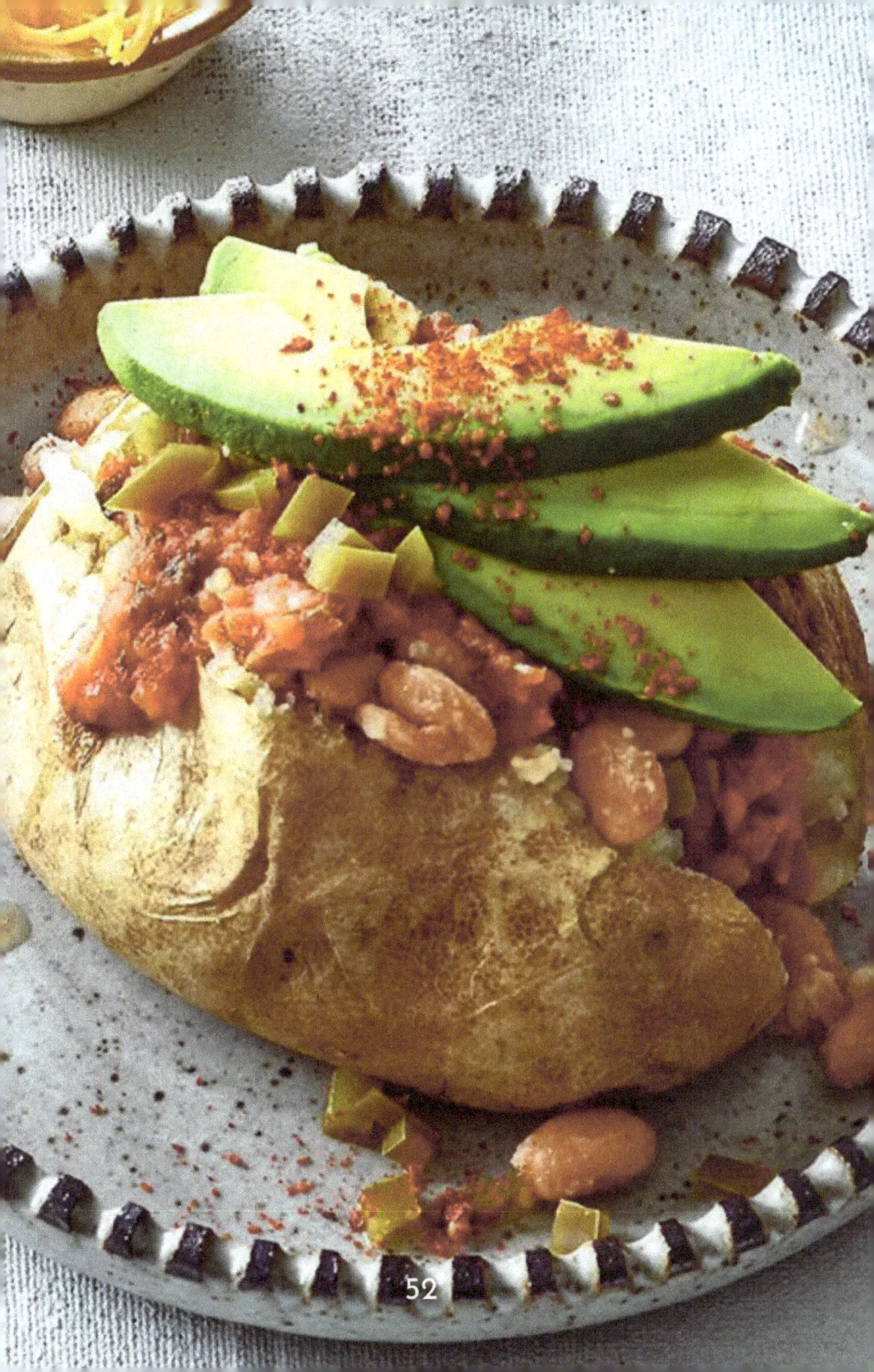

Grilled Shrimp Tacos

🍴 4 servings   🕐 20 minutes

INGREDIENTS

1 ripe avocado

1 tablespoon lime juice

1 small clove garlic, grated

¼ teaspoon salt

1 pound large raw shrimp (16-20 count), peeled and deveined

2 tablespoons salt-free Cajun spice blend

8 corn tortillas, warmed

2 cups iceberg lettuce, chopped

½ cup fresh cilantro leaves

½ cup prepared pico de gallo

DIRECTIONS

1. Preheat grill to medium-high.
2. Mash avocado with a fork in a small bowl. Add lime juice, garlic and salt and stir to combine.
Pat shrimp dry. Toss the shrimp with Cajun seasoning in a medium bowl. Thread onto four 10- to 12-inch metal skewers. Grill, turning once, until the shrimp are just cooked through, about 4 minutes total.
3. Serve the shrimp in tortillas, topped with the guacamole, lettuce, cilantro and pico de gallo.

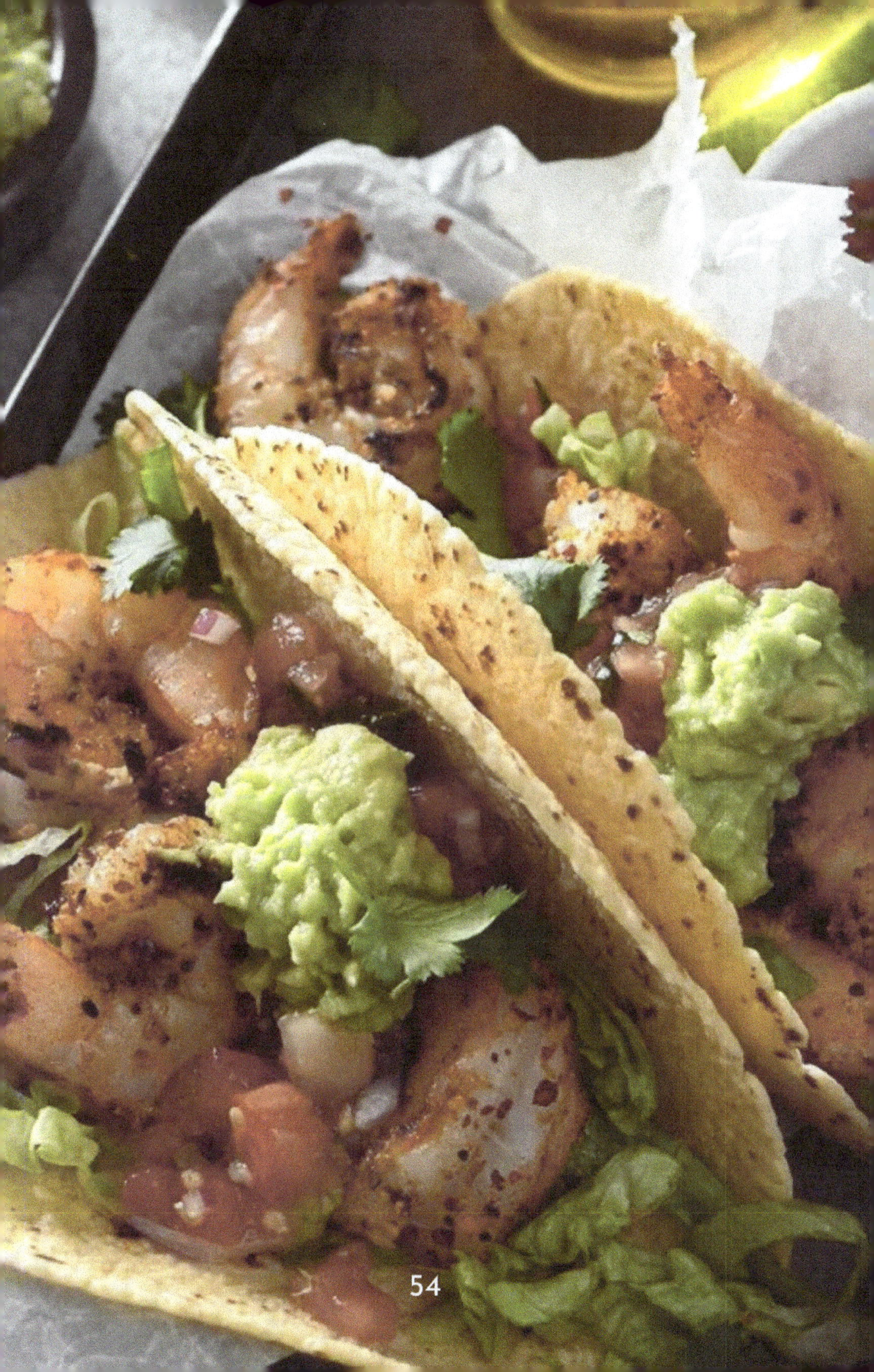

Baked Fish Tacos

With Avocado

🍴 4 servings   🕐 25 minutes

INGREDIENTS

1 tablespoon avocado oil

2 teaspoons no-salt-added Mexican-style seasoning blend

½ teaspoon salt

1 pound flaky white fish fillets, such as cod, haddock or mahi mahi, cut into 8 or 16 pieces

1 avocado, cut into 16 slices

½ cup pico de gallo

8 corn tortillas, warmed

DIRECTIONS

1. Preheat oven to 400 degrees F. Coat a large rimmed baking sheet with cooking spray.

2. Stir oil, seasoning blend and salt together in a medium bowl. Add fish and toss to coat. Transfer to the prepared baking sheet and bake until the fish flakes easily, about 10 minutes, depending on thickness.

3. To assemble tacos, place 1 or 2 pieces of the fish, 2 slices avocado and 1 tablespoon pico de gallo in each tortilla.

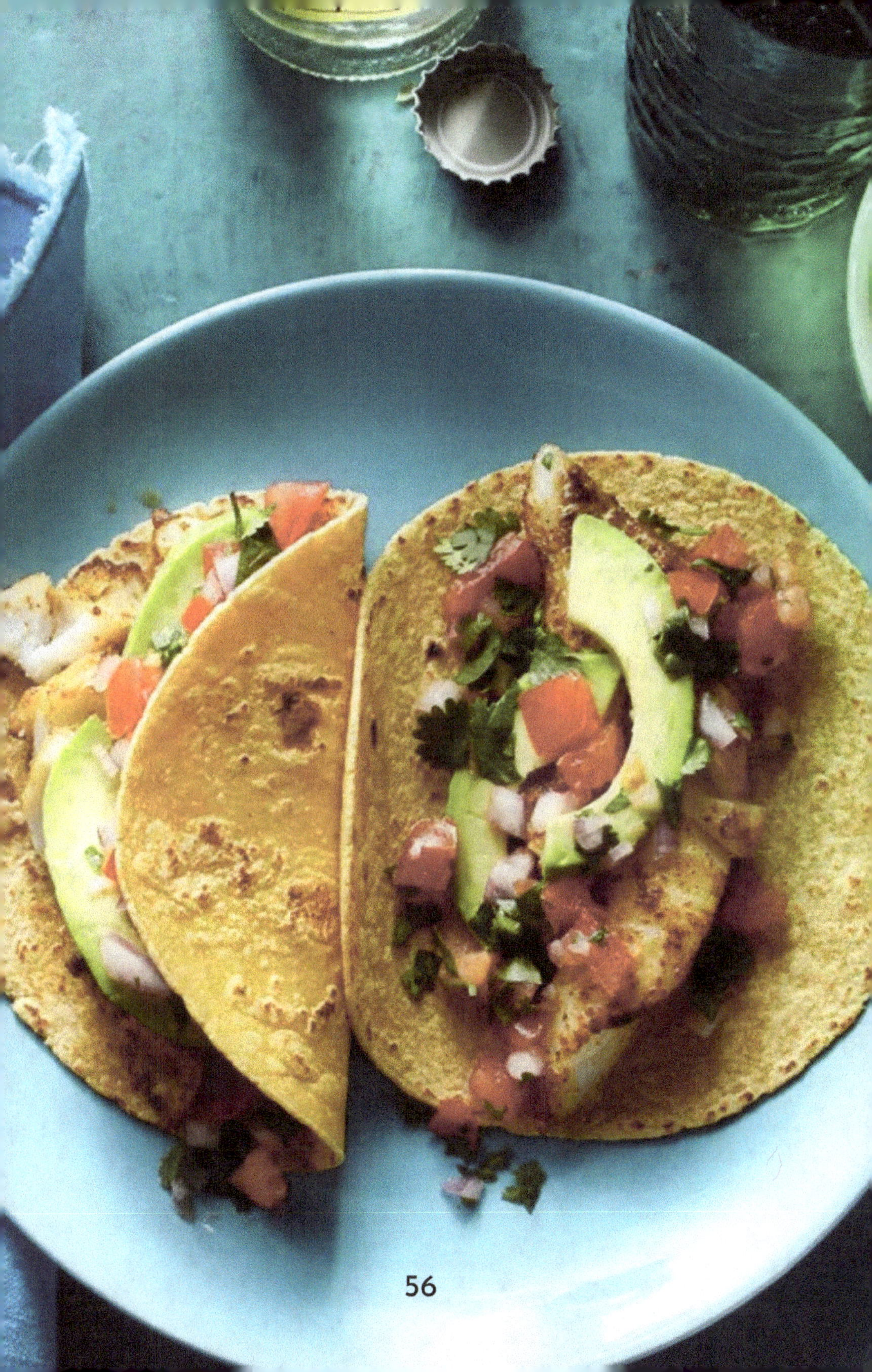

Red Beans and Rice

With Chicken

🍴 4 servings   🕐 20 minutes

INGREDIENTS

10 ounces skinless, boneless chicken breast, cut into 1-inch pieces

¼ teaspoon salt

¼ teaspoon ground black pepper

1 tablespoon olive oil

¾ cup coarsely chopped green sweet pepper (1 medium)

½ cup chopped onion (1 medium)

2 cloves garlic, minced

1 (15 ounce) can no-salt added red beans, rinsed and drained

1 container ready-to-serve cooked brown rice

½ teaspoon ground cumin

¼ cup reduced-sodium chicken broth

¼ teaspoon cayenne pepper

Lime wedges

1 pinch Cayenne pepper

DIRECTIONS

1. Sprinkle chicken with salt and black pepper. In a large skillet, heat oil over medium-high heat. Add chicken, sweet pepper, onion and garlic; cook and stir for 8 to 10 minutes or until chicken is no longer pink and vegetables are tender.
2. Stir beans, rice, broth, cumin and the 1/4 teaspoon cayenne pepper into chicken mixture in skillet. Heat through. Serve with lime wedges. If desired, sprinkle with additional cayenne pepper.

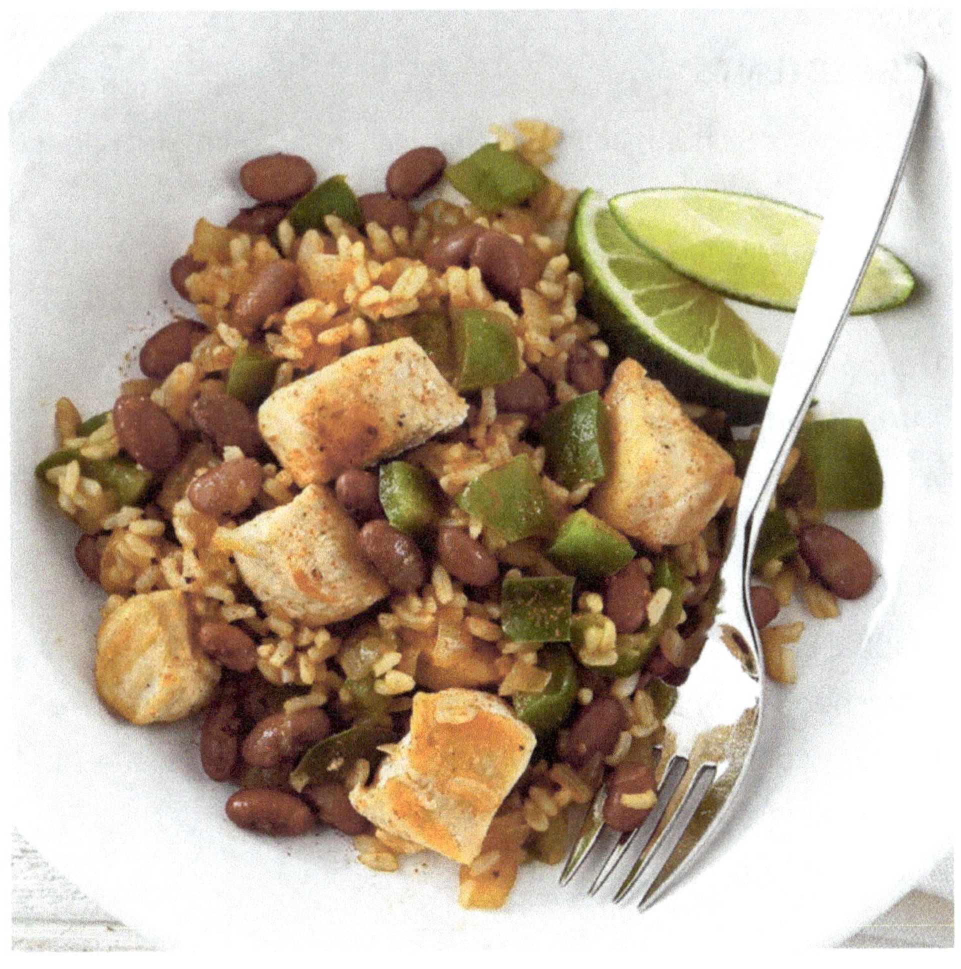

Sichuan Ramen Cup of Noodles

with Wilted Greens & Mushrooms

🍴 3 servings   🕐 25 minutes

INGREDIENTS

6 teaspoons Sichuan chile-bean sauce (toban djan) or chile-garlic sauce

6 teaspoons tahini

1 ½ teaspoons reduced-sodium vegetable bouillon paste

1 ½ teaspoons Chinese rice wine

1 ½ teaspoons packed light brown sugar

¾ teaspoon black vinegar (see Tip)

3 cups shredded napa cabbage

9 ounces extra-firm tofu, cut into 1/2-inch cubes (about 1 1/2 heaping cups)

¾ teaspoon Sichuan peppercorns, coarsely ground

1 ½ cups cooked black or brown rice ramen noodles (see Tip)

1 ½ teaspoons toasted sesame seeds

3 cups very hot water, divided

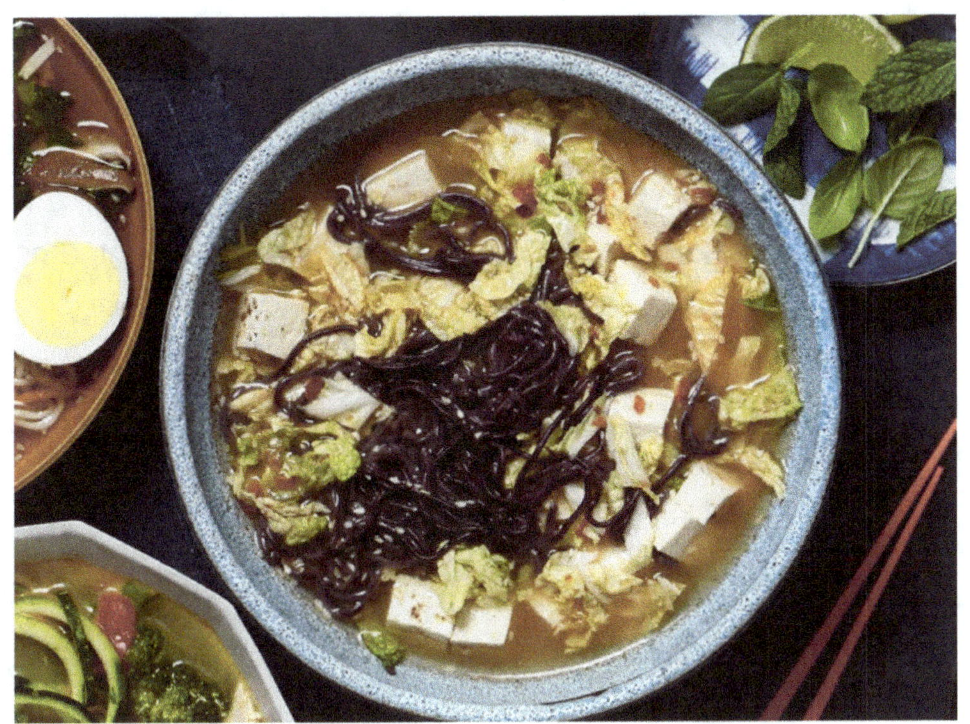

DIRECTIONS

1. Add 2 teaspoons each chile-bean sauce (or chile-garlic sauce) and tahini, 1/2 teaspoon each bouillon paste, rice wine and brown sugar and 1/4 teaspoon vinegar to each of three 1 1/2-pint canning jars. Layer 1 cup cabbage, 3 ounces tofu (about 1/2 cup), 1/4 teaspoon ground peppercorns and 1/2 cup ramen noodles into each jar. Top each with 1/2 teaspoon sesame seeds. Cover and refrigerate for up to 3 days.
2. To prepare each jar: Add 1 cup very hot water to the jar, cover and shake until the seasonings are dissolved. Uncover and microwave on High in 1-minute increments until steaming hot, 2 to 3 minutes. Stir well. Let stand a few minutes before eating.

Herby Fish
with Wilted Greens & Mushrooms

🍴 4 servings   🕐 25 minutes

INGREDIENTS

3 tablespoons olive oil, divided

½ large sweet onion, sliced

3 cups sliced cremini mushrooms

2 cloves garlic, sliced

4 cups chopped kale

1 medium tomato, diced

2 teaspoons Mediterranean Herb Mix, divided

1 tablespoon lemon juice

½ teaspoon salt, divided

½ teaspoon ground pepper, divided

4 (4 ounce) cod, sole, or tilapia fillets

Chopped fresh parsley, for garnish

DIRECTIONS

1. Heat 1 tablespoon oil in a large saucepan over medium heat. Add onion; cook, stirring occasionally, until translucent, 3 to 4 minutes.

2. Add mushrooms and garlic; cook, stirring occasionally, until the mushrooms release their liquid and begin to brown, 4 to 6 minutes. Add kale, tomato, and 1 teaspoon herb mix. Cook, stirring occasionally, until the kale is wilted and the mushrooms are tender, 5 to 7 minutes. Stir in lemon juice and 1/4 teaspoon each salt and pepper. Remove from heat, cover, and keep warm.

3. Sprinkle fish with the remaining 1 teaspoon herb mix and 1/4 teaspoon each salt and pepper. Heat the remaining 2 tablespoon oil in a large nonstick skillet over medium-high heat. Add the fish and cook until the flesh is opaque, 2 to 4 minutes per side, depending on thickness. Transfer the fish to 4 plates or a serving platter. Top and surround the fish with the vegetables; sprinkle with parsley, if desired.

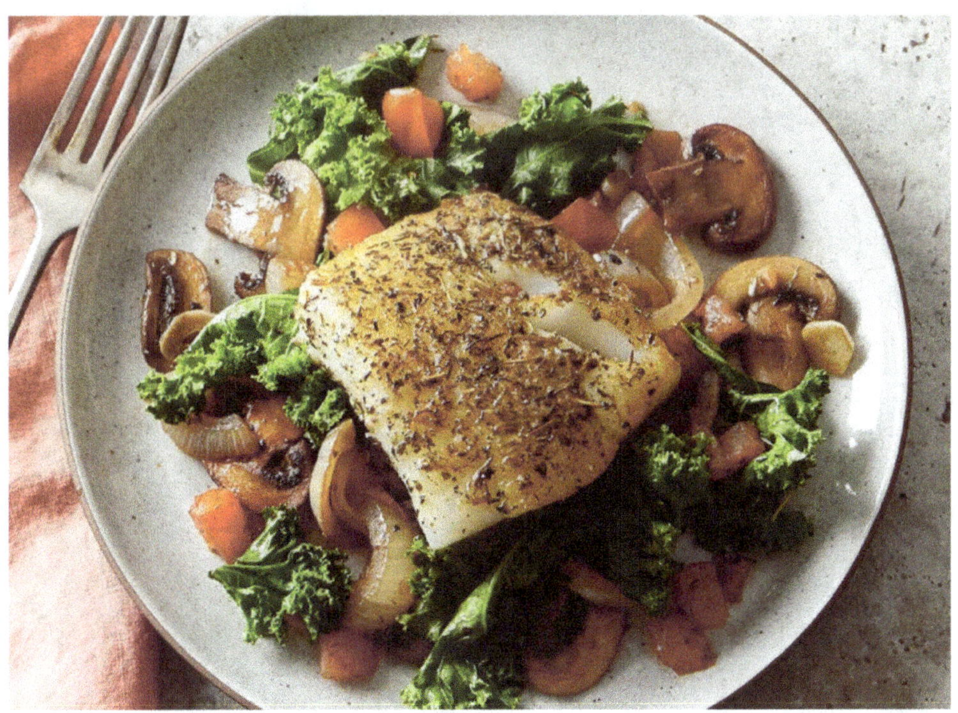

Grilled Salmon

With Cilantro-Ginger Sauce

🍴 4 servings   🕐 25 minutes

INGREDIENTS

Cilantro-Ginger Sauce

1 tablespoon toasted sesame oil

1 tablespoon fresh lime juice

1 tablespoon chopped fresh cilantro

1 teaspoon fish sauce

1 teaspoon minced seeded Thai red chile (about 1 large) or jalapeño pepper

1 teaspoon grated fresh ginger

1 teaspoon honey

1 medium clove garlic, mashed into paste

Salmon

1 pound skin-on salmon fillet (about 2 inches thick), preferably wild-caught, cut into 4 portions

1 tablespoon toasted sesame oil

½ teaspoon ground pepper

¼ teaspoon salt

DIRECTIONS

1. To prepare sauce: Whisk oil, lime juice, cilantro, fish sauce, chile (or jalapeño), ginger, honey, and garlic in a small bowl. Reserve 1 Tbsp. of the sauce in a separate small bowl to use for basting.

2. To prepare salmon: Preheat grill to medium-high (see Tip). Pat salmon dry with paper towels. Rub oil all over the salmon. Sprinkle both sides with pepper and salt. Place the salmon on the grill, skin-side up. Grill until the salmon lifts from the grates without sticking, about 6 minutes. Flip the salmon and brush with the reserved 1 Tbsp. sauce. Cook until the salmon lifts from the grates without sticking and flakes with a fork, 1 to 2 minutes more. Serve with the remaining sauce.

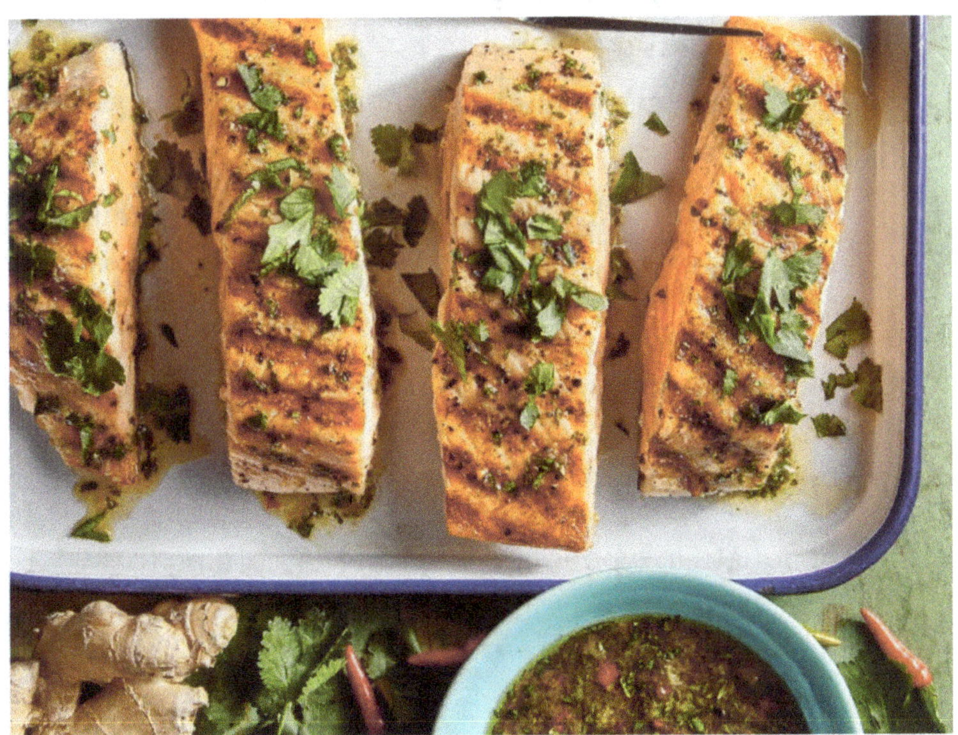

Classic Sesame Noodles

With Chicken

🍴 4 servings   🕐 20 minutes

INGREDIENTS

8 ounces whole-wheat spaghetti

3 tablespoons toasted (dark) sesame oil

2 scallions, chopped

1 tablespoon minced garlic

2 teaspoons minced fresh ginger

1 teaspoon brown sugar

2 tablespoons reduced-sodium soy sauce

2 tablespoons ketchup

8 ounces cooked boneless, skinless chicken breast, shredded

1 cup julienned carrots

1 cup sliced snap peas

3 tablespoons toasted sesame seeds

DIRECTIONS

1. Cook spaghetti in a pot of boiling water according to package directions. Drain, rinse and transfer to a large bowl.

2. Combine sesame oil, scallions, garlic, ginger and brown sugar in a small saucepan. Heat over medium heat until starting to sizzle. Cook for 15 seconds. Remove from heat and stir in soy sauce and ketchup. Add to the noodles along with chicken, carrots, snap peas and sesame seeds; gently toss to combine.

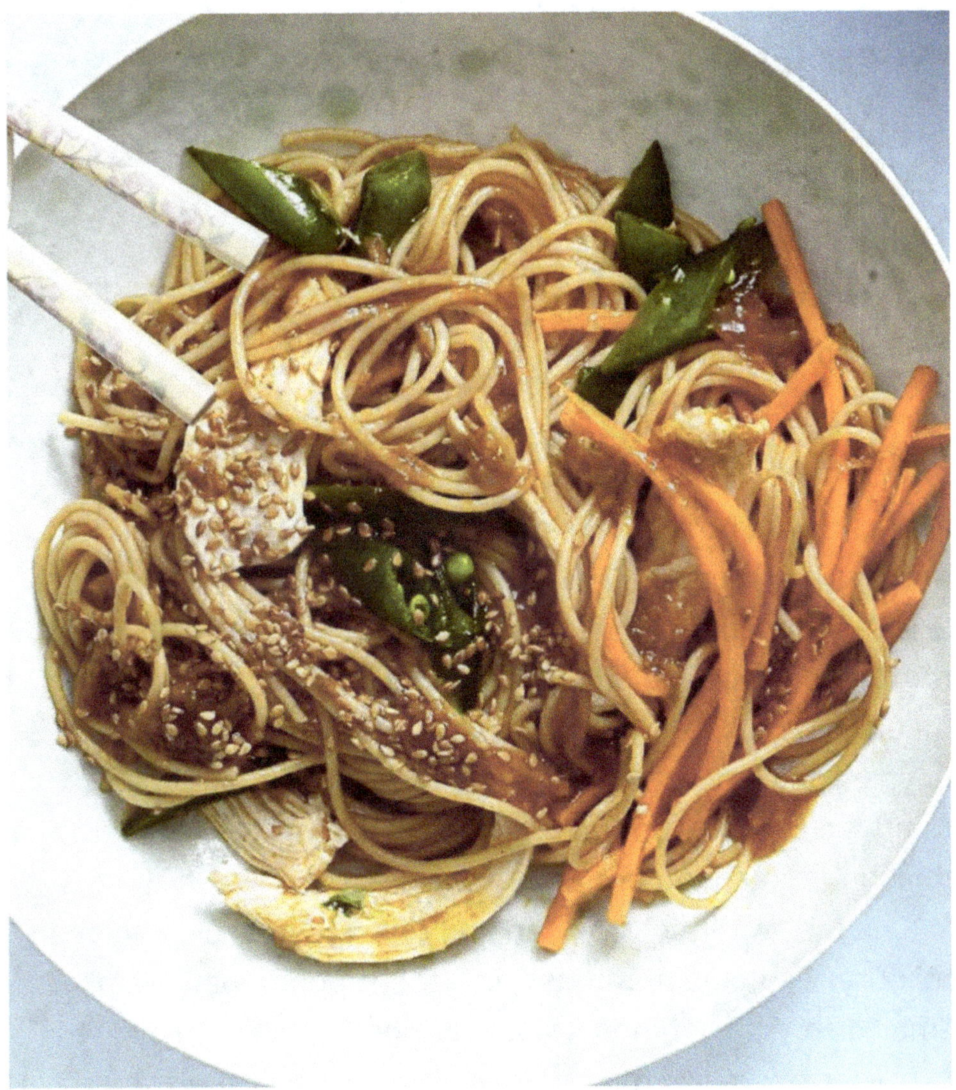

Stuffed Sweet Potato

with Hummus Dressing

🍴 1 servings   🕐 20 minutes

INGREDIENTS

1 large sweet potato, scrubbed

¾ cup chopped kale

1 cup canned black beans, rinsed

¼ cup hummus

2 tablespoons water

DIRECTIONS

1. Prick sweet potato all over with a fork. Microwave on High until cooked through, 7 to 10 minutes.

2. Meanwhile, wash kale and drain, allowing water to cling to the leaves. Place in a medium saucepan; cover and cook over medium-high heat, stirring once or twice, until wilted. Add beans; add a tablespoon or two of water if the pot is dry. Continue cooking, uncovered, stirring occasionally, until the mixture is steaming hot, 1 to 2 minutes.

3. Split the sweet potato open and top with the kale and bean mixture. Combine hummus and 2 tablespoons water in a small dish. Add additional water as needed to reach desired consistency. Drizzle the hummus dressing over the stuffed sweet potato.

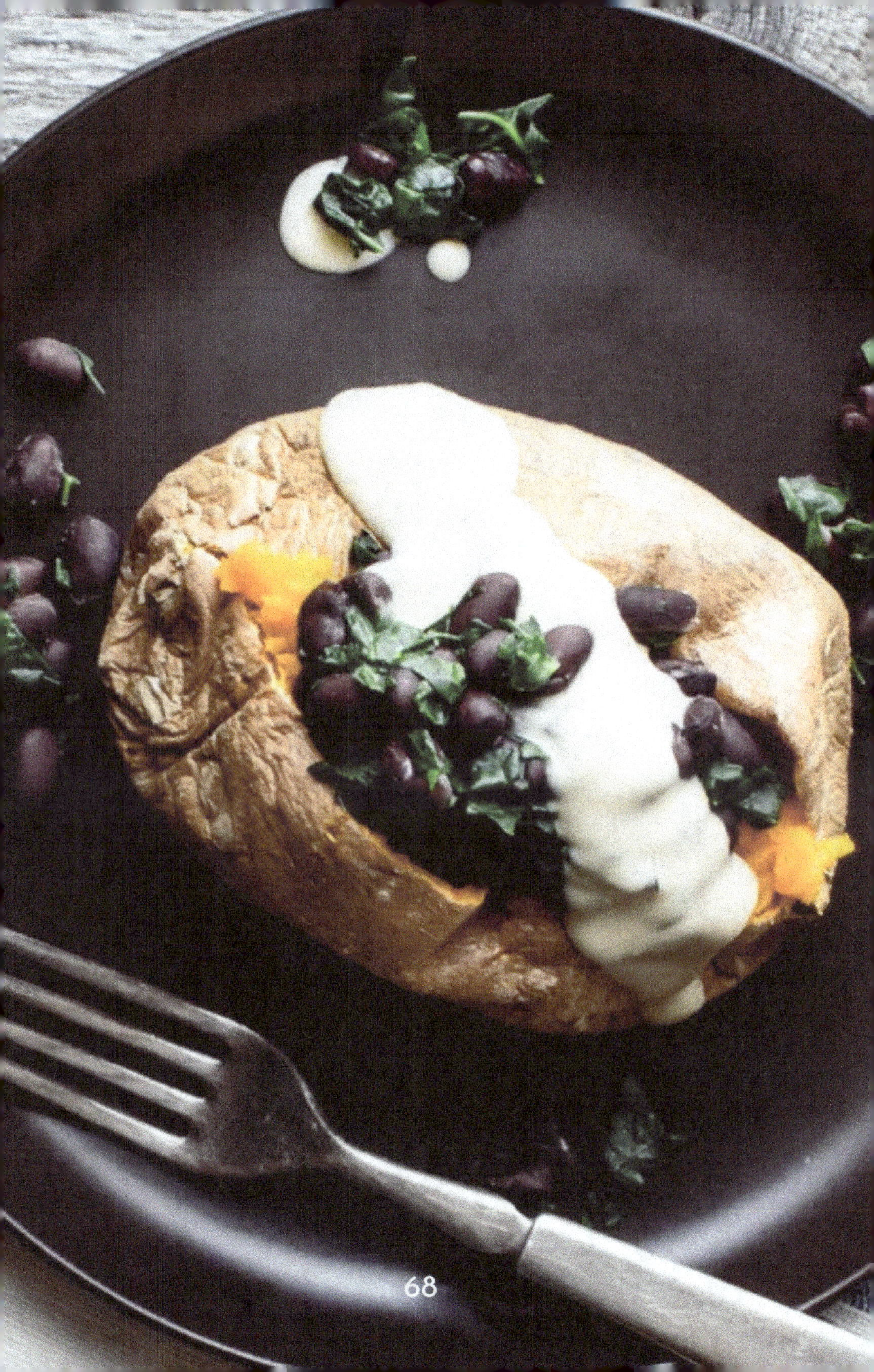

Ginger Beef Stir-Fry

with Baby Bok Choy

🍴 4 servings   🕐 25 minutes

INGREDIENTS

12 ounces beef flank steak, trimmed

1 tablespoon minced fresh ginger

1 ½ teaspoons reduced-sodium soy sauce

1 teaspoon dry sherry plus 1 Tbsp., divided

1 teaspoon cornstarch

1 teaspoon toasted sesame oil

2 tablespoons oyster-flavored sauce, preferably Lee Kum Kee
Premium

1 tablespoon vegetable oil

1 pound baby bok choy, trimmed and cut into 2-inch pieces
(about 8 cups)

3 tablespoons unsalted chicken broth

DIRECTIONS

1. Cut beef with the grain into 2-inch-wide strips. Cut each
strip across the grain into 1/4-inch-thick slices. Combine the
beef, ginger, soy sauce, 1 tsp. sherry, and cornstarch in a
medium bowl; stir until the cornstarch is no longer visible.

2. Add sesame oil and stir until the beef is lightly coated. Combine oyster-flavored sauce and the remaining 1 Tbsp. sherry in a small bowl. Set aside.

3. Heat a 14-inch flat-bottomed carbon-steel wok (or a 12-inch stainless-steel skillet) over high heat until a drop of water vaporizes within 1 to 2 seconds of contact. Swirl in vegetable oil. 4. Add the beef in an even layer; cook, undisturbed, until it begins to brown, about 1 minute. Using a metal spatula, stir-fry until lightly browned but not cooked through, 30 seconds to 1 minute more. Transfer to a plate.

5. Add bok choy and broth to the pan. Cover and cook until the bok choy greens are bright green and almost all the liquid has been absorbed, 1 to 2 minutes. Return the beef to the pan, add the reserved sauce, and stir-fry until the beef is just cooked through and the bok choy is tender-crisp, 30 seconds to 1 minute.

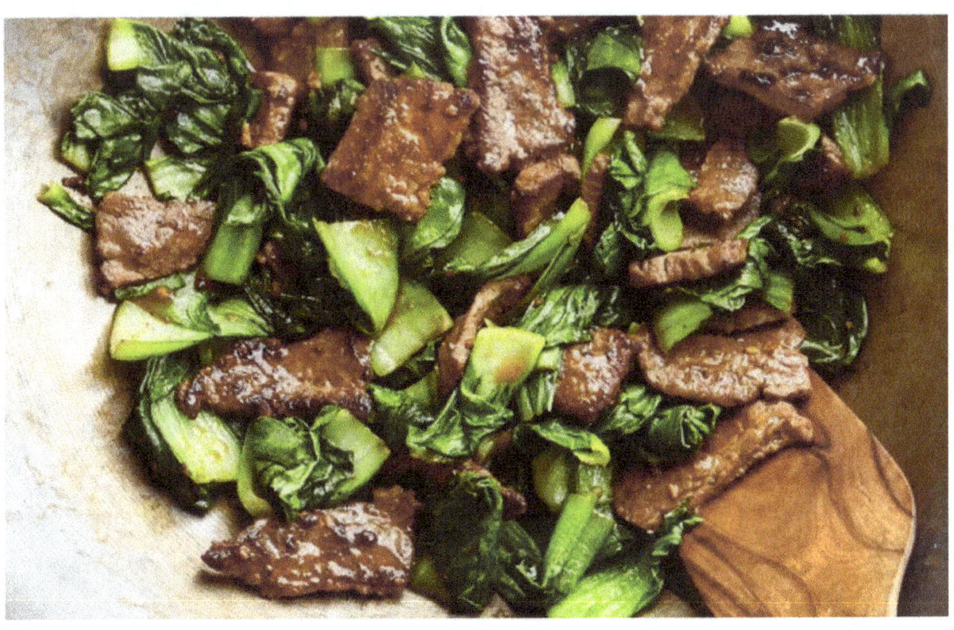